Hearing the Voice of People with Dementia

Opportunities and Obstacles

Malcolm Goldsmith

Hearing the Voice of People with Dementia

of related interest:

The Perspectives of People with Dementia
Research Methods and Motivations
Edited by Heather Wilkinson
ISBN 1 84310 001 0

Understanding Dementia
The Man with the Worried Eyes
Richard Cheston and Michael Bender
ISBN 1 85302 479 1

The Spiritual Dimension of Ageing
Elizabeth MacKinlay
ISBN 1 84310 008 8 pb

Including the Person with Dementia in Designing and Delivering Care
'I Need to Be Me!'
Elizabeth Barnett
ISBN 1 85302 740 5

Healing Arts Therapies and Person-Centred Dementia Care
Edited by Anthea Innes and Karen Hatfield
Series: Bradford Dementia Group
ISBN 1 84310 038 X

Spirituality and Ageing
Edited by Albert Jewell
ISBN 1 85302 631 X

Past Trauma in Late Life
European Perspectives on Therapeutic Work with Older People
Edited by Linda Hunt, Mary Marshall and Cherry Rowlings
ISBN 1 85302 446 5

The Social Construction of Dementia
Confused Professionals?
Nancy Harding and Colin Palfrey
ISBN 1 85302 257 8

Hearing the Voice
of People with Dementia
Opportunities and Obstacles

Malcolm Goldsmith

Jessica Kingsley Publishers
London and Bristol, Pennsylvania

First published in the United Kingdom in 2002
by Jessica Kingsley Publishers Ltd
116 Pentonville Road
London N1 9JB, England
and
325 Chestnut Street
Philadelphia, PA 19106, USA

www.jkp.com

Second Impression 1998
Third Impression 2002

Copyright © 1996 Malcolm Goldsmith
Preface Copyright © 1996 Mary Marshall
Extract from The Echoes Return Slow by R.S. Thomas
reproduced by kind permission of PAPERMAC
Extract from Counterpoint by R.S. Thomas reprinted
by kind permission of Bloodaxe Books Ltd.
The research on which this book was based was funded by the Joseph Rowntree Foundation

Library of Congress Cataloging in Publication Data

A CIP catalog record for this book is available from the Library of Congress

British Library Cataloguing in Publication Data

Goldsmith, Malcolm
Hearing the voice of people with dementia: opportunities and obstacles
1.Dementia 2.Mentally ill - Care

ISBN 1 85302 406 6

Printed and Bound in Great Britain by
Athenaeum Press, Gateshead, Tyne and Wear

Contents

For Jessie and Aubrey Smithers
with affection and respect

Wonderful examples

Preface

Dementia touches everyone. There can be few people in the more developed world who have not had some contact with dementia. In Britain perhaps nearly a million people have some degree of dementia and are struggling to remain part of families and other social groups whilst coping with their memory loss, their diminishing ability to reason and learn and their frequently high levels of stress.

Many of us have, or have had, relatives, neighbours or friends with dementia. Most of the care of people with dementia is carried out by relatives and friends at home. Staff working in almost any part of the health and welfare system will be working with people with dementia. A tiny minority are working in specialist domiciliary, day or long stay services for people with dementia. Most will be working with people with dementia alongside people with other disabilities. GPs, community nurses and home helps will have people with dementia on their caseloads. Staff caring for older people in settings such as geriatric wards and nursing homes will inevitably be working with some people with dementia. Most medical, surgical and orthopaedic wards will have some patients with dementia. Staff planning and managing services are having to apply their minds to meeting the needs of people with dementia throughout the health and social services.

Given the rapid increase in numbers there is an inevitable shortfall in expertise. Relatives, friends and staff are often learning as they go along without the benefit of lessons already learned by others. This book provides them with a starting point for an absolutely crucial set of understandings and skills: those relating to communication. It is based on a research study into how to hear the voice of people with dementia in the way that services are planned and run. It has become a book of wide interest to anyone who has been concerned at how little we know about the views of people with dementia. They are, generally speaking, silent. We do not know what people with dementia think about having dementia or how they think they can best be helped. We rarely ask them about their satisfaction with the services they receive as we would with other users of services. They rarely participate in decisions which are made about their care. This book is neither a conventional research report, nor a text book for staff. It is an unusual book in many senses: context, purpose, style, content and audience.

The context is unusual because Malcolm Goldsmith was a researcher for the Dementia Services Development Centre. This Centre aims to extend and improve services for people with dementia and their carers. It undertakes this task by providing a range of services for staff and volunteers including information, consultancy, training, research and publications. Researchers in the Centre are therefore part of a team committed to extending and improving services. Collecting and disseminating the latest thinking on any aspect of practice is the day to day work of the Centre.

Consumer participation in services is a fundamental plank of government policies. This was gathering momentum in the early 1990s and most health and welfare organisations were making strenuous efforts to involve users of services in planning and provision. There was increasing awareness too of the significant increase in the numbers of people with dementia; people who provide a real challenge to their families and to service planners and providers because their needs are so complex and constantly changing. Understandably the 'consumers' in this field were seen as carers and efforts were made to involve carers in the planning and provision of services.

The research behind this book was funded by the Joseph Rowntree Foundation, another organisation with a clear commitment to research as a means of informing policies and practice. The Joseph Rowntree Foundation has given priority to research into consumer participation in health and social services. It has funded substantial research into this issue and special studies focusing on particular client groups such as people with learning disabilities and carers. In 1993 it became clear that a neglected group was people with dementia, a group of people generally assumed to be quite incapable of such participation.

At this time we in the Dementia Services Development Centre were aware of a few people with dementia who were telling us what they felt. Robert Davis, a pastor in the USA, wrote *My Journey into Alzheimer's Disease* with his wife in which he vividly describes some of his difficulties and what help he most appreciated. Naughtin and Laidler in Australia included the views of several people with dementia in their book of experiences of several families (Naughtin and Laidler 1991). We were using this material in our training of staff and volunteers. We were also aware of people who had had an early diagnosis in memory clinics and were usefully sharing their views about their illness with staff. We were planning a major plenary on 'The Experience of Dementia' for the 1994 Alzheimer's International Conference because we had become convinced that there were techniques such as using the arts, psychotherapy and group work by which we could tap into this experience and that this understanding would improve our practice.

Reality orientation which was very popular in the later 1970s has been much criticised but it is important not to underestimate its contribution to changing the culture of care for people with dementia (Holden and Woods 1988). It promoted the idea that people with dementia can respond positively to changes in the way they are treated and to aspects of the physical environment. It opened the door to a great many new techniques such as reminiscence and validation therapy. Reality orientation was widely incorporated into regimes in long stay settings and led to an acceptance that communication was clearly possible and had therapeutic outcomes, although it was a fairly passive view of communication. Less accepted was the idea that people with dementia might have views about their experience of dementia, and about their preferences and the services they receive.

In October 1993 we submitted a project outline to the Joseph Rowntree Foundation. We claimed that 'In order to improve services for people with dementia and to make them more responsive to their individual wishes, it is necessary first to accept that people with dementia have a voice that is worth listening to, second to facilitate the use of it and third to hear it'. The project was funded and Malcolm Goldsmith appointed to undertake a literature review and a consultation exercise. The fact that there was so little written about the voice of people with dementia encouraged Malcolm to draw on a very wide range of sources.

The breadth of material in this book gives it an unusual richness. Scientific, psychoanalytic, religious and literary references mix with the feedback from a very substantial consultation exercise. Malcolm has elicited from his respondents an extraordinary amount of expertise which might otherwise have taken a long time to see the light of day. Although he himself is convinced that people with dementia can communicate if we have the skills to assist them and to listen, he also provides us with the opposite view and all the reservations.

One of the strengths of this book is that it is written for staff and volunteers rather than for an academic audience. It is a thoroughly good read. As such it is likely to be very influential. It will probably also be of great interest to family carers although they are not primarily the target audience. It will be of interest to a lay audience who are concerned about how little we know about the experience of people with dementia and the views of this very substantial number of people in our midst.

This book does not have the answers: it asks the questions, shares views and experiences and should generate further work and debate. Many of the respondents to the consultation exercise shared their feelings of isolation and their appreciation that someone was recording their experience. It is hoped that this book will be part of the process of giving them greater confidence in developing and sharing their skills.

There is a great deal to do before we can be confident that we know how to hear the voice of people with dementia. This book makes a contribution to changing the culture of dementia care and to ensuring that people with dementia begin to take their place as users of services with views of value to contribute to their nature and quality.

Professor Mary Marshall

Introduction

I would like to make three introductory points before the main text begins.

Methodology

I began this study by embarking upon an extensive literature search, looking particularly for issues relating to communication. Alongside this were six in-depth interviews with people with dementia and twelve less detailed interviews, together with many hours observing and sharing in the life of different types of caring facilities. There were four in-depth interviews with service providers and many discussions with other people involved in providing services.

Over one hundred people in key positions of service provision through-out Britain were requested to send names of people to be consulted and a Consultative Discussion Paper was sent to over a thousand nominated people inviting them to make comments. Over two hundred written replies were received and these were analysed and set alongside the issues coming from the literature review and from my interviews. In order to ensure anonymity and preserve confidentiality I have described the sources of the quotations I have used in general terms, although the replies to my document came from people who gave me quite specific job titles. I am grateful to the many people who responded to my invitation.

I was also fascinated to receive information coming from an Internet discussion on the subject, mainly conducted within the United States. Regular cross-referencing was made throughout the period of the study with my colleagues in the Dementia Services Development Centre at Stirling University, and the whole project was guided by an authoritative Research Advisory Group.

Terminology

I have used a large number of quotations, both from the literature in this field and from the many people who wrote to me following the circulation of my Consultative Discussion Paper. In all cases I have used the language and the terminology which they used. There is discussion about the 'politically correct' way in which to describe people who have dementing illnesses, and there is no universally accepted terminology. Working within the Dementia Services Development Centre I have accepted the convention in use there and prefer to use the phrase *people with dementia*. Other people talk about *sufferers* or *victims*, the *afflicted* or even the *demented*. I have reproduced whatever terminology was used in the original.

I have deliberately made no distinction between family carers and professional carers. In terms of the ability to hear the voice of the person with dementia or the possibility of communicating with them, the same or similar opportunities and obstacles face both, and I believe that the issues raised by this study are relevant to both.

Acknowledgements

My thanks are due to The Joseph Rowntree Foundation who generously funded this project, and particularly to Averil Osborne who guided it into existence. I have been warmly supported and questioned throughout by a Research Advisory Group which brought together a rich diversity of expertise and concern. Their critical participation has been vital. I am grateful to them for all their help, but it would be wrong to burden them with the responsibility for what has eventually been put on paper. What I have written are my own observations and conclusions, and I must take the blame for any mistakes or misunderstandings, although I hope that they are few in number and minor in detail. Members of the Advisory Group were:

Dr Lesley Jones, Research Support Worker, Joseph Rowntree Foundation

John Keady, Lecturer, School of Nursing and Midwifery, Bangor University

Sue Benson, Editor of Dementia Care

Harry Cayton, Director, Alzheimer's Disease Society

Martin Shreeve, Director, Social Services Department, Wolverhampton Metropolitan Borough Council

Derek Brown, Inspector, Social Services Inspectorate, Gateshead

Jim Manchester, Regional Manager Social Work, Westminster Care Limited, Devon.

I am also grateful to Professor Mary Marshall and to all my friends and colleagues in the Dementia Services Development Centre for their ongoing interest, support and stimulation.

Finally I would like to express my thanks to the staff of Jessica Kingsley Publishers who have produced this book in a very short space of time and with great courtesy and forebearance, and to Michael Kindred who compiled the index.

Malcolm Goldsmith

CHAPTER 1

The Echoes Return Slow

This chapter sets out the scene. It discusses definitions, different illnesses and some very general statistics.

It stresses the importance of communication and suggests that this can provide a new way into understanding. Confronting dementia can be a humbling experience, and perhaps we don't yet have adequate language to describe it.

> They keep me sober,
> the old ladies
> stiff in their beds,
> mostly with pale eyes
> wintering me…
> Some fumble
> with thick tongue for words,
> and are deaf;
> shouting their faint names
> I listen;
> they are far off,
> the echoes return slow.   (Thomas 1988)

A recent book suggested that working with people with dementia and their carers must be the most exciting field of social work to be in at the present time. It is high profile, it is challenging, it demands a multidisciplinary approach and it is open to new ideas and insights in ways in which so many other areas can only observe with a sense of nostalgia or envy. 'What other field has new models of services being tried all the time? What other field is so free from protocol and procedure that imaginative practice is still really possible?' (Chapman and Marshall 1993, p.1).

One of the areas that is currently being explored in dementia care is that of communication. To what extent is it possible to communicate with people with dementia? How much do they understand? How do they try to communicate with us and with others, and how do they understand and interpret our attempts to communicate with them? Problems relating to communication are two-way. There are problems experienced by the person with dementia and there are problems that we experience. Thus the opportunities for misunderstanding and poor communication are considerable. We need to find ways of encouraging and assisting them in their attempts to communicate with us and we need to ensure that we are doing everything possible to facilitate our own attempts to communicate. And all this needs to take place within a favourable context and environment.

Perhaps one of the first blocks to communication that has to be removed is the way in which we understand the nature of dementia. By building up a false picture of dementia we can then so easily go on to make assumptions that affect the ways in which we try to communicate, and may then greatly handicap our caring practices.

In 1992 the Michigan legislature in the United States passed a law making assisted suicide an offence. This followed publicity surrounding a Michigan pathologist, Dr Jack Kevorkian, who had developed a 'suicide machine' which he made available to people who were terminally ill and who wanted to die. In 1989 a young woman was diagnosed as being in the early stages of Alzheimer's and she made contact with the Michigan pathologist who did indeed help her to commit suicide. 'She was still able to speak quite coherently, and to play tennis. But she could no longer read a book, or read music and, when playing tennis, she had difficulty in keeping score. She knew that she might live another ten years or more, but that in the final phase, which can last for several years, she would be unable to recognise or communicate with anyone, and she would lie huddled in bed, her mind completely gone. She did not want to end her life that way' (Singer 1994, p.133).

Is that the only way to understand the approach of a dementing illness? Or are there alternative views which, whilst not denying the seriousness and horror of the illness, might provide other insights and possibilities which can serve to ameliorate the condition and open the door to possibilities that we have not thought of before? Questions about communication are at the heart of any such alternative exploration. In the pages that follow I hope to show that it is possible to approach dementia from a slightly different angle and that, by focusing upon issues relating to communication, a whole series of other questions and observations are raised. By taking these seriously our understanding of dementia, of what it is and what it might lead to, is challenged and developed. There is the need for us to hold together in a kind of creative tension the reality of the illness, as it inexorably progresses, with the reality of the person whom we know and love. In doing this we enter into a dialogue; ultimately it is a dialogue within ourselves. The nature of this dialogue has been uncannily described by the poet R S Thomas. Although his poem is not about dementia but about religious faith, it does in fact shed light upon our distress and dilemma when faced by the person with dementia:

> You show me two faces,
> that of a flower opening
> and of a fist contracting
> like the gripping of ice.
>
> You speak to me with two
> voices, one thundering
> on the ear's drum, the other
> one mistakeable for silence.
>
> Father, I said, domesticating
> an enigma; and as though
> to humour me you came.
> But there are precipices
>
> within you. Mild and dire,
> now and absent, like us but
> wholly other – which side
> of you am I to believe?   (Thomas 1990)

The general details about dementia can be picked up from a whole host of introductory texts. Dementia is not itself an illness. It is a syndrome, or group of concurrent symptoms, caused by a number of different illnesses. In common parlance the terms *dementia* and *Alzheimer's disease* are often used as though they were the same thing, which they are not. Dementia is the overall name given to a whole range of illnesses, the most common of which is Alzheimer's disease, where there is a gradual deterioration in the condition of the nerve cells in the brain. The second most common illness is multi-infarct dementia, sometimes called arteriosclerotic dementia. The brain is affected by an apparently random series of miniscule 'strokes' in which the blood supply to parts of the brain is cut off. Some people have both types of dementia concurrently. There is, as yet, no known cure for either condition. There are other less common illnesses which may also cause dementia, accounting for perhaps five per cent of all cases, such as Parkinson's disease,

Lewy body disease, Huntington's chorea, Creutzfeldt-Jakob disease, Korsak-off's syndrome (associated with alcoholism), persistent head injury and AIDS-related illnesses. The list is not exhaustive, but it illustrates the complexity of diagnosis, and this is something to which we return later in the book. It is equally important to stress the need not to use the term dementia for conditions or illnesses which, although sometimes presenting similar symptoms, are not actually produced by that cluster of diseases generally described as dementia.

Dementia is not a part of the normal ageing process, and although the incidence of dementia increases rapidly with age, even in the nineties it is still a minority of people who suffer from it. It is therefore important that we do not reinforce the popular view that dementia inevitably accompanies old age; it does not.

Table 1.1 The Age Distribution of People with Dementia

Age group (Years)	approx % of age group with definite dementia	approx % of age group not suffering definite dementia
60–65	0.7	99.3
65–69	1.4	98.6
70–74	2.8	97.2
75–79	5.6	94.4
80–84	10.5	89.5
85–89	20.8	79.2
90–95	38.6	61.4
95+	?	?
Total 65+	**6**	**94**

(These figures may considerably underestimate the number of people suffering from mild dementia, where diagnosis is more difficult).
Reproduced by permission of Churchill Livingstone from Alan Jacques *Understanding Dementia*.

It is clear that the incidence of dementia rises rapidly with age, but it is still a minority of people who are affected. However, with increasing numbers of people in older age groups, there is more likelihood that a greater number of families will have to face up to dementia at some stage or other. The approximate figures for Britain are these: out of a population of some 55 million people (9 million of whom are over 65 years old), there are between 5000,000 and 600,000 people with definite diagnoses of dementia. Possibly 15,000 to 20,000 of these are aged between 40 and 45. Approximately 200,000 to 250,000 are aged less than 80 and approximately 300,000 to 350,000 are aged over 80. It is notoriously difficult to agree upon figures

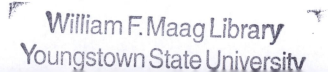

and different sources give widely differing figures. The ones given here are taken from Alan Jacques' book *Understanding Dementia* (1992).

The general population of 75–100 year olds contains a high proportion of women. As women have a longer life expectancy than men (78 years for women as opposed to 73 for men), and as more men were killed in wars than women, this means that amongst the people with dementia, the majority are women, and they are either widowed or single. There is no evidence to suggest that women *per se* are more likely to have dementia than men; the large numbers are attributable to demographic factors.

The vast majority of people with dementia live in the community, with something in the region of six per cent living in some form of institutional setting. Of those living in the community aged 85 or over, about 25 per cent of men live alone and about 50 per cent of women live alone – although, for the reasons mentioned earlier, the absolute number of women will be much higher than twice the number of men. Of those not living alone, they will be either living with their partner, with siblings or with their children. Because dementia is a progressive illness, many people will be diagnosed whilst living in one situation but, as time passes, they may need to move to other settings and may finish their days in some form of residential or nursing care.

The causes of dementia are, for the most part, still unknown. Certain forms may be related to alcohol abuse, to persistent head injuries or to AIDS-related conditions, but for the vast majority of people the causes are unknown. There are occasional and sometimes persistent theories, but the truth is that we still do not know. Many people refer to the use of aluminium pots and pans, but this has never been proved (or disproved!). A more recent idea linked Alzheimer's with the amalgam fillings that dentists use, but once again there is no proof. We do know, however, that it is not 'caught' from relatives, it is not sexually transmitted and cannot be passed on by using common cups and saucers and cutlery. It may seem obvious to state this, but such is the level of ignorance and confusion in the community that it is important to reiterate the point. Often people become aware of a problem after a sudden shock, bereavement or redundancy for instance but, again, there is little evidence to suggest that such dislocations have a causative effect. What often happens is that a change in circumstances, such as a bereavement, may bring to the surface certain behavioural, attitudinal or communicative problems that had been masked or unnoticed before.

Dementia is associated with memory loss. That is invariably the first thing that people think of when talking about the subject. But there are many other additional features to a dementing illness. Some of them are distressing in the extreme, even frightening for some people on occasion, but the great majority are not. Most of the time most people with dementia are relatively quiet and placid, ordinary people endeavouring to get on with their lives and make the most of the increasingly bewildering world in which they find themselves. Most of them are supported and encouraged by people who love them, and who try to accommodate to their forgetfulness and their some-times rather unusual behaviour. Bernard Heywood describes a typical little incident as he cared for his friend Maria:

> *4 September* Maria came down to say that one of her rings had been stolen and she asked me to go up, though I couldn't make out whether I was being accused or not…later, to my surprise, she gave me a costume jewellery ring that had one stone missing. I didn't want to take it, but she insisted.

> *5 September* Maria started talking about yesterday's rings. After a good deal of trial and error it transpired that she had given it to me to get the missing stone replaced, so that I could give it to Mrs Carstairs, as I'd said that I was going to marry her! I pointed out that Mr Carstairs was still around, but Maria said that she didn't think he'd live long and that when she'd asked me if I would marry Mrs Carstairs, I'd said yes. This is a supreme example of the awful language hazards. All I recollect is that once when she spoke about the Carstairs, she'd mentioned the word 'married' and I had thought that she was asking me if Mrs C was married to Mr C – I remember thinking that it was a surprising query – and I, of course, had said yes. Hence, apparently, her misunderstanding. This sort of thing is not only frustrating, but dangerous, and there must be many similar misunderstandings. To my relief, she took the ring back. (Heywood 1994, p.71)

It is because of instances like this, replicated a thousand times over, that the gulf between those with dementia and those who share their life seems to widen and widen, until a point is reached where many people say that it is impossible to communicate with them, or them with us. It does not require a great deal of imagination to conjure up a scenario of increasing isolation, bewilderment and frustration: 'I listen; they are far off, the echoes return slow'.

It is the argument of this book that, in far more cases than is commonly accepted, communication with people with dementia *is* possible. It is not always easy, and it can be a time-consuming and frustrating process, but it is a process well worth persevering with. The rewards are considerable, both for the person with dementia and for ourselves. There are certain skills which can be learned, there can be a sense of embarking upon quite an adventure, and there will also be a whole range of other issues opening up which may help us understand a little more and a little better the whole experience of dementia, and the love and devotion of so many carers, whether family members or paid professionals.

The poem by R S Thomas which I quoted at the beginning of this chapter continues with these words:

> But without them,
> without the subdued light
> their smiles kindle,
> I would have gone wild,
> drinking earth's huge draughts
> of joy and woe.

There is something about engaging with people with dementia which is very humbling. They draw us into a world in which we recognise the limitations of our own power and competence. We are forced to face up to parts of ourselves that we often prefer to remain hidden, and they invite us to respond to them in ways which take us by surprise.

It seemed appropriate that I should begin and end this opening chapter with poetry, for important though our professional skills and insights are, they are not totally adequate, they are not the final word. Poetry can often help us engage with 'facts' in ways which, without it, we could not imagine. Exploring how we communicate with people with dementia and how we hear their voice demands skills, understanding and insight. It also demands patience, love and poetry, for the echoes return slow.

CHAPTER 2

Hearing Views about Services

How do we know if the services that are being provided are appropriate – from the point of view of the person with dementia? The idea that they should be consulted is novel, and until recently has been dismissed out of hand. There is now growing evidence that such consultation is possible and six small studies are referred to.

Some of the opportunities or obstacles when we embark upon such a process form the basis for the remaining chapters in the book.

Setting out the context

For years mental decline in the elderly aroused little medical interest. Authorities in the first half of this century dismissed cognitive failure as an inevitable accompaniment of old age or due to incurable 'hardening of the arteries'. As a result the cognitively impaired elderly were left to languish in the back wards of hospitals and back verandahs of homes, while their problems, if recognised at all, were relegated to the back pages of medical journals.

After years of neglect, dementia in the elderly has suddenly become a leading topic in medical editorial pages. Many recent commentators have expressed their concern about the growing social importance and implications of dementia. Alzheimer's disease, the commonest cause of dementia, has thus been referred to as 'the silent epidemic', the 'coming deluge', 'one of the most pervasive social health problems of our generation', 'the fourth or fifth largest cause of death in the elderly', 'the rising tide', and 'the disease of the century'. (McLean 1987, p.142)

That is how Steve McLean, staff specialist in a psychogeriatric unit in Australia begins a long article on the problems of diagnosing dementia. He reminds us that, late in the day, medical and social concern is now taking dementia seriously. If it is true that the medical profession has been slow to respond to the challenge of dementia, it is also true that social and political concern for people with dementia has lagged behind the concern shown for many other marginalised groups within our society.

How do we know if the services that we are providing for people, particularly for people with dementia, are appropriate? How do we know if they are what the people themselves desire and need? In the Department of Health's publication *The Health of the Nation* it is clearly stated that everyone who provides or who purchases services has a duty 'to consult fully with users and their carers in the drawing up and monitoring of community care plans'. Furthermore, it adds 'they will need to ensure that service users are enabled to define their own health and social care to their maximum ability'. (Department of Health 1992)

Two years earlier, in 1990, the National Consumer Council had published a report which in one respect had seemed to state the obvious: 'in order to assess the effects of a service on the people who actually use it, a key starting point is to ask them – its consumers – which aspects of the service matter to them' (NCC 1990). But perhaps it was not stating the obvious, for there appears to be a widespread view, certainly in the case of people with dementia, that it is not possible to obtain their views on the services they receive or would like. The prevailing wisdom seems to be that the professionals, the medical, health and planning personnel, know best; and that it is best to leave things to them because they are more likely to know about the services available and able to comment upon them. In recent years this small group of professionals has been enlarged, and it is now very much more common to find that family carers are consulted – although even this is patchy and it is by no means universal practice. However, that the person with dementia himself or herself might also have a view on things seems to be a rather new and novel idea and one that is dismissed out of hand by a large number of people. Even Tom Kitwood, who provides some of the most stimulating and hopeful views in the whole area of dementia care, did not include hearing their opinions when he outlined his vision of a 'new culture of dementia care' at a conference in Bradford in 1994 (Kitwood and Benson 1995).

A report on residential care for elderly people with dementia published in 1993 by the Social Services Inspectorate began from the premise that 'all activities should start from a presumption that users can make decisions, exercise choices and live full and normal lives rather than they cannot do so' (SSI 1993, p.9). This is not to say that the reality and the seriousness of their illnesses were not acknowledged, but rather that the starting point should always be to focus upon what a person is able to do, rather than upon what they are not able to do. Also it assumes that, until proved otherwise, people are able to reflect on their situation and comment on the services they receive.

One person responding to my consultative document pointed out that there was a difference between people receiving services in their homes and those receiving them in residential settings. In her view this was a difference that was not sufficiently recognised and she wrote:

> I have a very specific and limited perspective from my recent experience of evaluating a case management service for people living in their own homes where I used a semi-structured interview with 95 people with dementia and their paid and unpaid carers, following them up over a year. One important point I would like to make is that I think there are going to be some crucial differences in the way one attempts to develop approaches to use with people living in their own homes compared to institutional populations. Furthermore, I think this is a neglected area needing more careful attention given the plethora of 'needs based assessments' for people with a wide range of stages of dementia in the community (in contrast to those in residential and day hospital facilities). Being in their own surroundings has many advantages and creates different dynamics and opportunities when attempting to hear their voice…I feel that there is a big difference in the perspective and experiences of carers working in a 'hands on' capacity and professionals with the 'hit and run' or 'monitoring' approach.

This project has not differentiated between the two, but it is a point which is worth bearing in mind. Perhaps those who are involved in care, whether in residential settings or within the community, might reflect upon how their particular context affects the process and possibilities of hearing the views of people with dementia.

There seems to be a detectable difference in the outlook of service providers between those who welcome the expression of choice and comment, and those who assume that their understanding is somehow better or more accurate than that of those who receive their services. They work on the assumption that it is not possible to obtain consumer feedback. Of course, this assumption is not new, and it is perhaps the prevailing experience of most people who are in receipt of services, irrespective of their illness or disability, that their views do not count. This point has been forcibly made by Jenny Morris who wrote:

services should facilitate the expression of choice, and in this way people would be empowered to achieve a quality of life; instead we have a history of service provision based on so-called 'experts' expressing choices on our behalf. It is this silencing of our voices which disables us rather than our physical, sensory or intellectual impairments. (Morris 1993)

A similar point was made by a manager who wrote to me saying:

This is a much neglected area...there will need to be a huge shift necessary in organisational culture before the decision makers begin to listen to people with dementia – they are finding it hard enough at the moment to listen to service users who are articulate and confident.

Consultation and choice are closely linked to issues of power and control and, as we shall see later, a sense of powerlessness is one of the abiding feelings that communicates itself when talking with people with dementia. This will be looked at in greater detail in Chapter 5. Tim Booth movingly describes the difficulties of trying to obtain the views of people in residential accommodation, and he portrays a world in which powerlessness and dependence exist side by side.

The net result is that either residents' views are considered unreliable and treated with suspicion or when asked, residents are found to have very little to say. (Butler 1990, p.163)

The situation for people with dementia is that few people take either the time or the trouble to ascertain their views. This is presumably largely because they think that the nature of their illness means that self-reflection and expression are rarely possible, and also because to attempt it is often a slow and laborious task. However, recognising that it is difficult is not the same thing as saying that it cannot be done. As Mary Winner pointed out, the key issue is not 'whether these users' views are important, but how indeed we might equip ourselves better to understand and obtain them' (Winner 1993, p.8).

Dementia inevitably brings with it problems of memory, short stretches of concentration and problems with assembling words, but these things do not in themselves mean that communication cannot take place. They mean that greater care has to be taken, and that the process may take longer than at first envisaged. It is the argument of this book that great numbers of people with dementia, even in advanced states, who are not thought able to communicate, actually have a great desire to do so. It is for others to acquire the skills which will enable them to understand and interpret the experiences and views of those who struggle to make themselves heard.

Some evidence

It is strange to reflect that the commonly held view is still that people with dementia are unable to comment on the services they receive or their experiences of them; and yet when studies have been made to test out this view they all seem to indicate otherwise. Of course, the studies are few and the number of people involved is small. Nevertheless, where research has been undertaken to see whether the views of users of services can be detected, they have all come up with interesting insights and positive recommendations.

In 1990 two clinical psychologists, Laura Sutton and Felicity Fincham, worked on a study to find out how people with mild to moderate communication difficulties viewed and experienced the respite care service they received (Sutton and Fincham 1994). Using a process of interviews which were open-ended and client-centred, and close observation, they were able to build up a 'Life Plan' matrix (a model that comes from the field of learning difficulties and mental disability). What emerged was that all the people in the study expressed a preference to be in their own home, but they were often aware that they needed to be in respite care for the sake of their carer. It was clear that it was the *social* rather than the *physical* aspects of care which were of greatest importance to them. The researchers were able to get a general sense of whether people saw the services in a positive or negative way. The people spoke about their enjoyment of being entertained, their dislike of sitting around doing nothing, 'just waiting', and the fact that they liked being out of doors and going for short walks. The research showed that the people with dementia could 'share with us their experience of the care they are receiving in the here and now. Indeed, they provided a remarkably rich account which, we felt, was not coloured by a "need to please", or a sense of gratitude…in other words, we were getting something of the lived experience of those receiving respite care'. By acknowledging the ability of many people with dementia to communicate verbally, there is an implied acknowledgment of the need for staff to develop the appropriate listening skills, which of course applies to all service providers, and to recognise the crucial importance of interpersonal as well as environmental influences on people's well-being. As the authors conclude, it 'cautions against the all too ready assumption that dementia sufferers are too confused or out of touch with reality to offer a users' perspective'.

In the same year Lynne Phair published a study in which she interviewed clients who came into contact with the services being offered at a particular centre (Phair 1990). She recognised that many people might be uncertain about obtaining the views of the 'elderly confused', but the study showed that the clients 'both mentally alert and mentally frail, were able to give their perceptions' of the unit. 'It is fundamental for a democratic society', she claims, for it to 'devolve power to the ordinary citizen as far as possible and with psychiatric patients in particular, [an] consumer involvement helps to reduce negative feelings'. She then widens this conviction to ensure that the mentally confused are seriously considered in her own research project.

> 'Gaining opinion from confused elderly people can sometimes cause anxiety and...some authors feel that it is not appropriate to gain opinions from elderly demented people. However, they do have a role and as they are the consumer they do have the right to express their feelings and views about services that they are receiving [because] the perception of the clients...may actually be different to those of the carers and those giving the service' (Phair 1990, section 1–4).

In 1993 David Sperlinger and Louise McAuslane undertook a pilot study of the views of users of services for people with learning difficulties and dementia in one of the London Boroughs (Sperlinger and McAuslane 1994). They began by recognising that for those providing services, the difficulties in obtaining the views of users about those services can seem to be insurmountable. They found that a literature search threw up few examples. The authors of this study were concerned with the practical methods of obtaining the views of people with learning difficulties and with understanding the experiences of people with dementia. They hoped to find a way of approaching people with dementia which would enable them to say something, both about their experiences and themselves, in order that the researchers could make some proposals as to practical methods of obtaining a clearer picture of their views on the services they were receiving. That may sound a rather convoluted approach but it serves to illustrate just how novel the idea is that we should hear the voice of people with dementia. We do not yet have a clear idea about how we should go about this exercise, and so Sperlinger and McAuslane's piece of work is in fact a very helpful and innovative preparatory approach.

They interviewed in depth six people in the early stages of dementia and the interviews were recorded and subsequently analysed. For four of the six people it became clear that there were issues, concerns and worries that they were anxious to share with the researchers, and these kept cropping up throughout the interviews. Although many of the questions in the interviews were about the more physical aspects of care (travel, food and the environment, etc.), the things that seemed to be of more concern to the users were the *social* aspects of care. Even when the people interviewed were unable to give clear responses to the questions, the researchers found that 'it was still usually possible to get a general sense from most of them of whether they saw the services in a positive or negative way' (Sperlinger and McAuslane 1994, section 6.3, p.10). Although the study was limited in its size and scope, it does indicate the potential value of seeking the views of people with dementia about the services which they use, and shows that it can be done. The authors conclude, 'our experience suggests that generally people using these services have plenty to say...it is clear from this pilot study that it is possible to consult with some users of the dementia services in a meaningful way', and they go on to outline how more systematic surveys might be taken in the future' (Sperlinger and McAuslane 1994, section 7.5, p.10).

In 1994 the steering committee of the local Alzheimer's disease society in Sutton approached the Psychology Department of the St. Helier NHS Trust with a view to carrying out a consultation with both users and carers involved with a Weekend Break project. The study, by Jessica Lam and Lynn Beech, gives more strength to the view that it really is possible to engage with people who have dementia and discuss their experience of, and views about, the services which they receive. They conducted twelve interviews with users of the project, and these demonstrated that people with dementia were able to express their views and concerns, and that they were able to indicate whether or not their needs were being met. The users showed a high level of awareness of the impact that their difficulties had on relatives and carers.

The authors summarised the consultation by saying that

> the interviewees expressed high level of insight into the concerns, worries and feelings of responsibility experienced by members of their families who were caring for them...participants were also acutely aware of their difficulties in expressing themselves clearly, they evidently felt greatly frustrated and distressed by this at times. (Lam and Beech 1994, section 5)

Once again, the users were far more concerned about the social aspects of the service than they were about physical considerations. The need to belong, the desire for companionship, the need to feel valued and the desire to be engaged in stimulating activities or those which aroused pleasant memories were the concerns which surfaced time and time again. Lam and Beech concluded that 'despite a progressive decline in memory and cognitive powers, people with dementia retain the capacity to experience the whole range of emotions, and the capacity to contribute to, and benefit from social relationships' (section 5).

A study by Brenda Gillies focused on the subjective experience of dementia, but had some interesting comments to make on service provision. She undertook semi-structured interviews with 19 people with dementia, and also with their carers. The majority of subjects were interviewed once, but six people with dementia had second interviews. In spite of a general lack of understanding (albeit acquiescence) about *why* they attended the services they did, this group of subjects expressed considerable satisfaction. Commonly staff received universal praise for their kindness and attentiveness and the subjects were able to specify particular features of day care they enjoyed, including the social company, singing, dancing and quizzes and 'therapy'. Where there appeared to be fewer activities the responses were less positive. Another interesting factor which she discovered was that, even bearing in mind the positive response people gave to day care, they were 'unwilling to increase their participation and guarded their autonomy in choosing how often they attended' (Gillies 1995, p.12).

Keady, Nolan and Gilliard have written about their work in interviewing six people with dementia and their family supporters. They argue that 'if we are to achieve the ideal of responsive, flexible, individually-based services for people with dementia, we must listen carefully to their experiences and their opinions' (Keady, Nolan and Gilliard 1995, p.15).

Some reflections

If the conclusions reached by people who have researched this field are that people with dementia are able to reflect on their experience, and if they are also able to have views on the services they receive, and are able to communicate these – then why does the idea of hearing the views of people with dementia still seem so novel?

When I began my own piece of work on this subject, many people told me that I was wasting my time. Others were not quite so blunt but looked rather quizzical and came up with comments like 'Oh, that will be interesting, I would like to know how you make out', whilst a few others gave me a great deal of encouragement and support. It was as though there were three set positions. The first was that people with dementia cannot be understood, and they need to have decisions made for them – the 'we know best, poor things' approach. The second was that although in theory it was a good idea to hear their views, it really is not practical, but it is good that we hold on to the concept. The third view was a sort of gut reaction that it *must be possible* somehow, and that we need to keep working away at it until we find a way through. These three positions or viewpoints become quite obvious when the literature is surveyed, or when service provisions are observed.

I began by undertaking six in-depth interviews with people with dementia. These were tape recorded and subsequently written up and analysed, followed by twelve less formal interviews. I was interested in analysing not only the content of these interviews, but also the process and my own reaction to it. Where I found things difficult, I was interested to explore why this was so. To what extent were some of the problems of communication my own problems rather than the problems of the person with dementia, and to what extent did the very process and the 'mindset' that I brought have an effect upon the communicative relationship? I became quite fascinated by these rather philosophical questions, and began to wonder if there could be value in opening up a range of questions which might help us to have a fresh look at the ways in which we communicate with people with dementia, and identify some of the problem areas – actual or potential.

Ten areas of concern emerged, and these were set out in a brief consultative discussion paper. This was sent to more than 1000 previously identified people, who were concerned about issues relating to hearing the voices and the views of people with dementia or with providing services (not that the two are necessarily different!). More than 200 written responses were returned, and this book is the result of merging these views from the 'front line of practice' with ideas and insights which emerged in the literature search. I found that there were some fruitful areas of debate waiting to be explored further.

We are not yet in a position to be able to speak easily with people with dementia, but we do know that *some* people seem to be able to communicate with *some* people with dementia. The challenge is – how can we enable *more* people to communicate *more easily* over a wider range of topics with *more* people with dementia?

CHAPTER 3

Is There Anyone in There?

We know so little about the experience of dementia. This chapter sets out some of the tension between the biomedical and social approaches – but both are necessary. The concept of personhood is introduced. Accounts of the experience of dementia are discussed. We are left with the unresolved question as to whether there is still a 'person' remaining as the illness advances, or does the very notion of dementia destroy what makes someone a person?

What happens to a person when they suffer from a dementing illness? We know that there are different forms of dementia and that these affect the brain in different ways. We know that something physical is happening within the brain, and that there is a deterioration – usually slow, but not uniformly slow. We know that a person's ability to remember is affected – not only their ability to remember events and names and faces, but also their ability to remember what things are for, their ability to remember how to behave in socially accepted ways, and their ability to remember how to decode the messages that come from the brain which may be telling them that their bladder is full, or that they have just eaten, or that it is night outside, or that it is cold. Different people are affected in different ways, and the way in which the illness presents itself might be quite different for different people. Nevertheless, there is a recognisable pattern of deterioration, but what else is happening?

Is it death by degrees? Is it a living hell? Has the person that we knew before disappeared? Do they know what is happening? Is there more to dementia than a medical diagnosis and a slow slide into death? Do we know what is going on in a person's mind – in their very being?

Our knowledge about dementia is still rather basic, and understanding about the many aspects of the subject is not developing at the same speed or with the same degree of insight. This means that occasionally there can be a lack of tolerance between people approaching the subject from different starting places. To put it crudely, there exists a certain tension between what might be called the *medical approach* and the *social approach*. It is not that they are mutually exclusive, and both would want to stress their need for the other, but they have developed along different routes and sometimes it is difficult for them to speak the same language, or to understand the concerns of the other. We need both and there is need for both aspects to advance. They are not in competition with each other but, for a variety of reasons, there is often the temptation to maximise the importance of one and to minimise the contribution of the other. Which one is promoted and which is dismissed depends to a large extent upon where you are standing, and what you are doing.

The questions posed here are not easy to answer. They tend to be philosophical, even religious in their scope. But they are real questions, and ones which people ask time and time again.

What is going on? Is there still a real person in there? For some people, the conclusion they reach is that the person they knew has long since died, even though they still breathe. For others, they believe that they can detect signs of uniqueness and personality long after other people have become wearied through trying. Are we imposing personality from without? Or denying it when it is still there? What is happening when, for long stretches of time, there appears to be no insight or understanding and then suddenly a coherent sentence or an incisive observation is made?

A biomedical approach

The strictly 'medical' interpretation has been spelled out quite clearly by Fontana and Smith in an article on 'unbecoming' (Fontana and Smith 1989). They claim that in the early stages of the disease people with dementia continue to interact on the surface 'as if they were sentient beings' whilst what is actually happening is that they are losing the rational part of their self and relying on deeply embedded forms of sociability in order to carry them through social situations. During these early stages people give the appearance of normality, but what is actually happening is that this 'self' that they are presenting is becoming 'increasingly devoid of content'. It is, they say, 'unbecoming a self'.

According to this view, and this is the way in which they describe it, the self of the person with Alzheimer's disease slowly begins to deteriorate as the disease attacks the mind until, in the end, the individual becomes totally unaware of his or her surroundings. The person experiences increasing bodily deterioration until there is a total loss of mental functioning, and death. It is a bleak picture which they draw. Their observations, they say, indicate that people seem able to cling on to their social constructs, and so they are able to operate within company until a very late stage of their illness. These instinctive reactions outlive others and should not be thought of as demonstrating that they continue to understand. We are left with the job of 'filling the gaps', that is, of making coherent the rather jumbled messages that come through to us. Fontana and Smith (1989) call this 'normalising competence' and they say that it is an important task when dealing with people with Alzheimer's disease because they seem to be able to retain the 'form' of much social behaviour but the content of their actions becomes increasingly meaningless.

> For Alzheimer's disease patients what remain to the very last, beyond unique individual expressions, are the social routines that create and maintain a sense of self and acceptance of that self by others. The self of Alzheimer disease patients appears to consist mainly of internalised social norms and customs that are presented to the world, and of basic emotional needs – a need for attention and love from others, and a close world of egocentrism and selfishness...

> ...the self has slowly unravelled and 'unbecome' a self, but the caregivers take the role of the other and assume that there is a person behind the largely unwitting presentation of self of the victims, albeit in reality there is less and less, until where once there was a unique individual there is but emptiness. Witnessing as the 'other', the 'unbecoming' of self, creates a feeling of emptiness in the caregivers' hearts. Thus, they act as agents for the victims and impute to him or her the last remnants of self (p.45)

This approach is also followed in one of the most popular and respected books on dementia, a book which gently guides our thinking and gives a most illuminating survey. In *Understanding Dementia* Alan Jacques (1992) takes the hypothetical case of an elderly lady who shows no evidence of any thoughts or feelings, who seems to have no understanding and no speech left. Anything which she does understand, he says, will be quickly lost.

> It is most unlikely that such a patient is 'locked in' with lots of thoughts and feelings that she cannot express, as can happen to people who suffer severe speech disorders or severe Parkinsonism. It is much more likely that there is very little mental activity at all and that she is living in a world of fragmented experience, a world of meaningless sights, sounds, smells, tastes and bodily sensations, partly experienced

consciously and unconnected to her equally fragmented emotions and activities.

We can have little conception of what those fragmentary sensations or thoughts are like, or what a fragmentary emotion is…what we can be sure of, I think, is that the experience for the onlooker is different from the experience for the sufferer. The onlooker sees the decline, the emptiness of the patient's mind, her inability to do anything for herself, her disintegrating personality, and so may feel a sense of loss, of pessimism, of boredom, of degradation. The patient herself, on the other hand, is unlikely to be aware of or feel any of these changes in a coherent fashion. She will not recall all the things that she used to be able to do and so she will not be able to recognize the change in herself. She will not be able to feel the humiliation of her dependent position. She will not sense the passage of time. Or she may experience the wrong feelings, or jumbled bits and pieces of feeling, some appropriate, some not… Our feelings about what is good or humane for a very severely demented patient cannot come from an understanding of what she feels as an individual, or of what she 'wants'. These concepts are meaningless and so any real understanding is impossible. At the final stages the patient may be assumed to have no real subjective awareness, no sense of self at all, and to be in this sense mentally 'dead'. (p.172)

Jacques goes on to stress that although we may not be able to understand a person, nor they us when they reach these advanced stages, we must not assume that we cannot understand the earlier stages. The problem seems to be how to differentiate between these different stages and when to conclude that the person has 'unbecome'. There is a real danger that, in order to protect ourselves, we distance ourself from the person with dementia thereby compounding the losses that he or she is already experiencing. This process of distancing is one about which quite a number of people have written. To adopt a stance which relies heavily on this *medical* approach is understandable since it helps us to keep distress at bay. As Kitwood and Bredin (1992) commented:

Professionals and informal carers are vulnerable people too, bearing their own anxiety and dread concerning frailty, dependency, madness, ageing, dying and death. A supposed objectivity in a context that is, in fact, interpersonal, is one way of maintaining psychological defences, and so making involvement with conditions such as dementia bearable. (p.270)

Personhood

In recent years there have been attempts to approach dementia from different perspectives and notable among them is the concept of *personhood*, developed and propounded by Tom Kitwood and others. Whilst not denying the contribution of medicine, he argues that we need to have a fundamental shift in the way in which we approach the subject. Instead of seeing 'a set of deficits, damages and problem behaviours, awaiting systematic assessment and careful management' (Kitwood 1993a, p.16) which effectively turn the person into an object, he says that we need to work on the basis of seeing the person as a whole. This does not deny the presence of a dementing illness but sets it within a context which is social rather than medical. We should understand a person's dementia as being the result of a complex interaction between their personality, their physical health, their biography or life history, their social psychology (the network of their social relationships) and their neurological impairment (the actual dementing illness). All these factors combine to make a person who they are, and to concentrate on one of the factors only without proper regard for the others is to treat the person as less than a whole person.

A Church of Scotland minister who has Alzheimer's disease now lives in a residential home. His condition has slowly deteriorated over the last few years but an essential 'spark' remains. A friend recorded in poetry the experience of visiting him.

> The wilderness within you has been stripped;
> only the graininess is left.
> Yet so much intact,
> despite erosion of that sense of self;
> so much remaining
> which can cross the chasms
> when words get in the way of knowing
> – a touch, a smile –
> with your engrained benevolence
> you make me mindful of what humanness entails.
> You have no cogent thought, and yet
> your muddled words
> are full of thoughtfulness.
>
> I sing for you, and wonderfully
> you join in, add harmony.

Then shall the tongue of the dumb sing;
for in the wilderness shall waters break out,
and streams in the desert.
I feel as Moses must have felt
striking the rock.   (De Luca unpublished)

Using the concept of personhood in dementia care can breathe a sense of hope and new life into an area that has so often been seen and experienced as totally negative and full of foreboding. Pessimism used to pervade the whole subject and images such as 'a living death' or 'death that leaves the body behind' were common descriptions. The personhood approach is an attempt to reinstate the person with dementia as a living person who happens to have a particularly distressing illness, rather than the 'victim' of a psychiatric illness. Comments such as 'the brains of these people are virtually dead. All they need now is quietness and basic physical care' are seen as being much less than the whole truth, and determined efforts are being made to think more positively and to look for grounds of hope rather than to dwell on the inevitabilities of decline.

In a radio discussion between the psychiatrist Anthony Clare and the writer and broadcaster Michael Ignatieff, the latter says:

> I learned as much from my mother when she couldn't speak to me, when she couldn't communicate, when she simply stared and received our kisses on her cheek, as I learned when she was joking and laughing. What she taught me was that it's just an illness. It's a terrible illness, but it's just an illness. And there's life beyond the illness. (*All in the Mind*, BBC 1994)

This expresses the tension between the medical and the social models. Of course there is an illness, often terrible in its consequences, but people are more than their illnesses, and an overreliance on the biomedical viewpoint can rob us of appreciating the subtleties and complexities of a person in their personal and social context. There is more to a person than that. As Karen Lyman, pointed out in an important article (1989) 'in reality, the psycho-social experience of a dementing illness cannot be contained within biomedical concepts of brain disease' (p.600).

It is interesting to note that this questioning of an overreliance upon the biomedical approach is taking place in a wide range of services. Nursing, for instance, is being urged to take the psychosocial seriously. Edith Hillan, writing about nursing elderly people with dementia, recognises that for many years nursing practice was based upon this biomedical approach where 'the patient is seen as a repository of disease emitting signs and symptoms from

which a diagnosis could be made and appropriate treatment prescribed'
(Hillan 1993, p.1890). She went on to admit that nursing paternalism was
the norm, particularly with elderly people who were too weak or confused
to refuse all the washing and exercise that they were forced to receive. A
similar sort of reappraisal can be seen in literature in the field of occupational
therapy (Peloquin 1993a, b). An increasing number of nursing homes and
residential homes are now writing about their experiences in trying to base
their work on the principles of personhood, as illustrated by these reflections
from a nursing home in Bradford:

> In their despair, relatives often assert that dementia has destroyed their
> loved one's personality and that he or she is no longer the same person.
> It is easy to see what they mean, yet as time goes by, given the right
> help and support, the person does start to regain 'selfhood'... We
> would like to challenge the commonly held misconception that in
> dementia personality is permanently and irretrievably destroyed...
> Given the opportunity, people with dementia are able to function as
> valuable members of their social group and they have the potential to
> regain control over their own lives. The stumbling block to achieving
> this may well be our limited conception of what is and what is not
> possible for them...our experience has prompted us to re-examine our
> prejudices about the nature of selfhood and personality in those who
> have dementia and to ask ourselves if we are perhaps holding them
> back from fulfilling their true potential...damage to personhood is
> normally attributed to the effects of dementia. However it is clear that
> enormous damage is also caused by the negative attitude to which
> people with dementia are exposed... Are we being unrealistic and
> idealistic in proposing that, given the right environment and support,
> a person can embark on a personal voyage of rediscovery and be
> helped to undertake a search to regain his or her selfhood? (McGregor
> and Bell 1993, p.29)

The crux of the issue seems to be quite simple. Either we go along with the
view that the very nature of the disease means that the person with dementia
gradually 'unbecomes', and there is little that we can do to arrest this process
or make much meaning of it. Or we take the view that the medical condition
is but part of the process, and whilst that may well be serious, there may still
be ways of rediscovering and maintaining personal identity. Now, of course,
these two positions are somewhat exaggerated, but nevertheless there does
seem to be a basic divide in the stance or approach which most people take,
albeit unconsciously. We are not in a position to be able to 'prove' one and
'disprove' the other. It seems that ultimately it all boils down to almost an

act of faith! We seem to have a gut reaction that somehow and somewhere there is life to be sustained and nurtured, or we have a gut feeling that the person is disintegrating as a 'person', and although there are ways in which we can care for them which may be more sensitive and humane, in the end there is little that can be done in terms of reaching them as a recognisable, unique human being. I would not want to encourage people to see one approach as 'right' and the other as 'wrong', but rather to recognise that in this complex area there may be good reasons why some people veer towards one and others veer towards the other. The important thing for us is to keep our minds open and to be ready to acknowledge that there is much that we do not yet know, and we must always be prepared to be taken by surprise and realise that our stance can only be, at best, provisional. There is clearly need for further exploration and training here as we seek to explore our gut reactions and hold in balance the inbuilt tensions of such an approach.

I am persuaded that the approach argued by Tom Kitwood has much to commend it and that we need to pay a great deal more attention to the social dimension before we conclude that there is little that we can do in terms of communication and interaction. As Kitwood (1990a) says:

> If dementia is simply the result of an ineluctable process of degeneration in nervous tissue, as the 'standard paradigm' implies, then changing the social psychology would have no radical effect on the course of the affliction. If, however, a dialectical account is nearer the truth, we may expect some surprising outcomes when the social psychology is changed. (pp. 194–5)

This 'dialectic' involves a dynamic relationship with other people, with the environment, with that which is outside of and beyond the person with dementia. If it is true that the condition of the person can be affected by these relationships, and that this can be for good or ill, then it becomes very important that we understand our own role. Sabat and Harre have argued that if a person with dementia is to sustain his or her part in the social world, then other people are required (Sabat and Harre 1992). Often these other people do not contribute what is required and needed, but when they do 'get it right' and when they provide the stimuli or the support or the affirmation that is required then 'some personae can be sustained by the dementia sufferer and self, in this sense, is not lost'.

Kitwood and Bredin (1992) put it beautifully:

> The dementia sufferer needs the Other for personhood to be maintained…the Other is needed, not to work with growth, but to

offset degeneration and fragmentation: and the further the dementing
process advances, the greater is the need for that 'person work'...the
self that is shattered in dementia will not naturally coalesce; the Other
is needed to hold the fragments together. As subjectivity breaks apart,
so intersubjectivity must take over if personhood is to be maintained.
(p.285)

Betty Davis (1989) wrote in the epilogue to her husband's book *My Journey
into Alzheimer's Disease*:

Death would be better than this – to hold on to the box when the
present is used up – hoping the box can bring again the joy of the
reality of the gift – but the box is empty! This is what one has to look
forward to with Alzheimer's disease. The body of the one you love –
devoid of all expression, of recognition, of joy – here but not here.
You are destined to live with the memory of who he was. How do you
prepare for the holocaust? (p.159)

Is there no other way? Have we no words of hope or comfort for someone
experiencing such grief and desolation? Has the present gone entirely out
of the box or is it still there and might there be ways of accessing it, of seeing,
touching and experiencing it? It is to meet such questions as these that so
much work is now being done to explore what actually happens to the
'person' with dementia, and to see how far communication is still possible.

The experience of dementia

The following short poem was written by a sixty-nine year old woman who
was diagnosed as having Alzheimer's disease six years previously:

> This day is mine
> I've yet to know tomorrow
> I'll use it well
> For who can tell
> If joy will come or sorrow.
> What was can be no more
> What is can be today
> I'll use the day for all it's worth
> Before it too will fade away.   (Helen 1994)

As yet there are few subjective accounts of the experience of dementia,
although the number is growing reasonably quickly. The book referred to
earlier, *My Journey into Alzheimer's Disease* by the American evangelical clergy-

man Robert Davis (1989) was perhaps the first attempt to describe what it was really like. He described the confusion and fear that he experienced:

> It is very painful to go into crowds. When I sit in the middle of a large audience, I find myself becoming more and more panic-stricken, and quite often I will leave the church service, confused and completely drenched with sweat. I do not enjoy large crowds, and I can barely keep up with the people that I meet in the stream of people without becoming confused and having to sit down and regroup my thoughts... In other places, such as shopping centres with uneven lighting and crowds of people moving in all directions at once, I become confused and completely lost...headaches are a common occurrence. Whether they are caused by emotional disturbance or organic problems I do not know. I do know that in times of emotional stress I have tremendous headaches that produce confusion and finally produce physical exhaustion. At the end, my mind blanks out, and I become unresponsive and uncommunicative. (p.104)

The other significant book, written by someone with Alzheimer's disease is Diana Friel McGowin's *Living in the Labyrinth* (1993). A former legal assistant and freelance writer, she makes it clear that people with Alzheimer's disease (certainly at the stage she is at when she writes) still have memory, are able to relearn things that they have forgotten, and have both good days and bad. She writes passionately that we need to find ways of enabling people to live with the disease by helping them to focus on their strengths and capacities rather than on their losses and their illnesses.

There are an increasing number of accounts of the experience of dementia now being written which offer some insight into what it must be like for the person. It is still rather like a patchwork quilt at the moment – a whole series of discrete accounts which we set alongside each other without too much concern for any overall, unifying pattern, but enormously valuable nevertheless. A typical example comes from Scotland. A journalist interviews Min, a fifty-one year old woman and hears how she views her illness:

> Well in some ways it wouldn't be so bad if I didn't know what was happening...now I have to face the prospect of my mind going while I'm still physically healthy and full of energy...the driving means everything to me. It's always represented my personal freedom...I know that sometime I'll have to stop and that will be total hell...I know that there is going to be a time when I have to be taken to the loo, and put to bed and all the rest, and I don't want him (her husband) doing that. It's not the kind of life I want for either of us. Sometimes

you see people being wheeled about, apparently in a dream, and you wonder if they know what is going on inside. I don't want that for me or him and I feel that now is the time I ought to be making these kinds of decisions. How can you decide later when you've lost the power of making decisions? (Wishart 1990)

These are some of the issues that will be discussed in later chapters, but for the moment the important thing is to realise that there is a time when many, if not all, people are aware of what is happening to them. What we do not know is for how long this period lasts. The conventional wisdom seems to be that there comes a time when people are unaware of their situation, as described in the biomedical approach discussed earlier. But an increasing number of people are now raising questions about that and suggesting that it might be the case that people are aware of their situation far longer than we had previously supposed but, because of their fears initially and then their difficulties in communication, they do not express their awareness. This is one reason why it is so important that we discover ways of communicating better and longer with people who have dementia. Opinion on the matter is divided, but some people such as McGregor and Bell (1993) have 'an absolute conviction that people with dementia retain insight into their condition to a far greater degree than one would imagine. This insight continues right until they die and can often be the cause of deep, yet unrecognised depression' (p.30).

Cohen (1991) in an interesting article points out that although a great deal of research has helped us to understand the physical and emotional costs to carers of looking after people with dementia, very little has been done on the subjective experience of the person who is ill. Although we now know much more about cognitive changes in dementia, we still do not know much about how individual people adapt emotionally and cognitively to progressive degenerative brain disorders. The net result of this is that we have not therefore developed sufficiently the psychological, behavioural and family therapeutic interventions that might be possible, and this means that we might not be providing the best care. We are at risk, he says

for not delivering adequate care to our patients and their families. If we do not get to know our patient's experience of the illness beyond the results of medical, cognitive and functional tests and assessments, our clinical decisions will not represent patient needs equitably in the caring transactions that occur. (p.7)

Cohen goes on to argue that, at least until the late stages, people with Alzheimer's disease can still display the qualities of faith, hope and 'the will to live and love'. In a phrase which I have seen quoted elsewhere he speaks of one person having described living with the disease as 'living in a dustbowl of hope as well as an oasis of despair', but he says it was important to her to be a participant in life for as long as possible. Success was 'playing the game, not winning it' (p.7).

He also describes the experience of another person:

> Having Alzheimer's Disease made me face ultimate realities, not my bank account. My money, job and other parts of life were trivial issues that restricted my growth, my spiritual growth. Alzheimer's Disease transferred me from what I call the trivial plane to the spiritual or personal plane. I had to face the absolute horror of the A word, and I began a dialogue with my existence, a dialogue with my life and my death. (p.9)

Cohen hopes that as our knowledge of their subjective experience grows, so we might have more accounts written by them; more poetry and pictures from them and, echoing words which could have come from Kitwood, he concludes that 'the existence of catastrophically and chronically ill people compels us to discover what it means to be human' (p.11).

Alison Froggatt (1988) comments on the fact that there seems to be much more knowledge about how the experience of dementia affects family members and carers than about how it affects the person with the illness – 'it is part of the incipient ageism in our society that it is easier to identify with the carers than with the sufferers' (p.131). She then describes how close observation and discussion with people identified as having a dementing illness show that, certainly in the early stages, people have some insight into and awareness of what is happening to them. The question is, is it possible to continue to explore that experience and can the person continue to bear the pain of holding onto the reality of his or her world, and of reviewing their past experiences and memories? The answer seems to be that most people can. Indeed, there is evidence that people positively want to hang on to what they know and value and appreciate the attempts of people to help them do so, as the work of John Killick (1994) demonstrates. He works with people on a one-to-one basis, writing down for them as much as they can remember about their past and what they feel and think about their present. Apart from anything else, he says, it helps to confirm their individual worth at a time when circumstances have reduced their choices dramatically.

It is a slow and often heart-rending process but the response has been remarkable and, over time, most of these people seem to recognise – and appreciate – the attempts to help them 'get in touch' with their real selves. Tears may run down their cheeks as they comprehend, even momentarily, what they have lost. Yet they still have much to give.

But we must also act upon the knowledge gained to ensure that we do not forget that each person has a history, a personality and an approach to life that is unique. I would suggest that there is more infringement of liberty in proceeding as if this were not so. (p.10)

Foley, in a chapter entitled 'The experience of being demented' comments that there still persists in some quarters the 'unfortunate misperception that the demented person is unaware of the fact of dementia' (Foley 1992, p.30). She describes different grades of severity of intellectual loss, disturbance and affect, and points out that people will respond to the stresses of the environment in different ways but that there are some generalisations which can be made about what people with dementia think and feel.

- Some people will have a full awareness that something is wrong with their intellectual capacities and they will retain some sense of awareness throughout the duration of the disease.
- Some people seem to have no awareness of any deficiency in their intellectual state, and they act accordingly, even though their world is disintegrating around them.
- Others, aware that something is wrong, strenuously deny it and set up schemes 'of rather transparent concealment', convincing themselves that their denial is successful in fooling others.
- Most common is the far less clear-cut, more changeable pattern whereby many people have clear insight at the beginning and then lose it, finishing up either without any awareness or with a highly developed denial system in place. Depending upon the circumstances, the variations in intellectual capacity and awareness may be in terms of weeks or days – or sometimes the fluctuations can be down to hours and minutes.

The strange thing is, and no one seems to know why this is so, that some people in even rather advanced states can have moments of clarity and recall which allow their normal or former personality and intelligence to emerge for just a short time before again being swallowed up. Sometimes a person may have gone weeks or months without making any coherent conversation when, suddenly, they speak and demonstrate an awareness of their situation which takes the carer completely by surprise.

In a study of six people in the early stages of dementia Keady, Noland and Gilliard (1995) observed that:

> ...each of the interviewees provided an open, honest and deeply moving account of their feelings. From these accounts of living with dementia, it would appear that the description of this experience as a journey – largely, it should be added, into the unknown – is very apt. Indeed, in listening to these accounts, it was apparent that in truth, despite professional background and experience, we know very little about the experience of dementia and the perspectives of those who live with it. (p.15)

In 1985 Cohen, together with a colleague Eisdorfer, described six phases of change experienced by people with dementia (Cohen and Eisdorfer 1986). They suggested that people might be able to learn how to cope with some of their problems if they knew what to expect. Developing work done in other areas by Elisabeth Kubler Ross they set out the stages of dementia:

(a) recognition and concern;

(b) denial;

(c) anger, guilt and/or sadness;

(d) coping;

(e) maturation, and

(f) separation from self.

These stages, they felt, provided people with a conceptual framework which might help them to sustain a self-awareness and to evaluate, understand and respond to their own needs and feelings during the different stages of their illness.

Well, is there anyone in there? I detect in the literature quite a divide between the detached and rather clinical assessment and approach and the more engaged and exciting approach. Both have strengths and both have weaknesses, but at this stage it is far from certain whether we can answer unequivocally that 'Yes, there is someone in there'. However, to deny that possibility leaves us with a daunting and bleak future. In this context, the words of Michael Ignatieff make a great deal of sense:

> One of the strongest impulses in writing about Alzheimer's Disease is to make it (and it's an odd thing to say) intellectually interesting,

because I believe passionately that we can only have compassion for what we feel interested in. As long as senility was regarded as one of those tragically incomprehensible but essentially boring things that happen to old folk, we didn't get to grips with it. In fact Alzheimer's is an illness which has an absolute fascination because it takes us to the roots of the self...when somebody gets Alzheimer's – are little bits of memory falling away to the kind of aggregate process in which more and more of the memory gets lost? – or is it something very different which is happening, in that the person is forgetting who it is that is doing the remembering – is the person forgetting *themself* first, and then the memories go? (*All in the Mind*, BBC 1994)

CHAPTER 4

Different People are Affected
in Different Ways

People have different personalities before they develop dementia. There are different illnesses which cause dementia. So there are many variables that have to be taken into consideration. There is a general recognition that we need to see people as individuals, but it is not always easy to to provide individualised services, and so there is often considerable frustration -- for carers, service providers and for the people with dementia.

Too often people are grouped together, just because they have a diagnosis of dementia.

Because people are different there is a need to develop flexible, specialised and person-centred care.

It is a truism to say that no two people are the same. The differences between people are legion. It is also true that when people develop dementia the illness affects them in different ways. Indeed, since there is no specific illness called 'dementia', we are therefore dealing with very different people being affected by one or more of a number of different illnesses. In the consultative document which I sent out I wanted to explore this area of 'differentness', and in it I suggested that:

> it has been argued that dementia is the result of a complex interaction between personality, biography, physical health, neurological impairment and social psychology. Lumping people together under the label of 'dementia' and approaching them in the same way is likely to increase the problems of communication and make it more difficult for us to hear their voice.

Variables to take into consideration

Of course before people become ill they have developed their own unique personalities. Some people have been 'larger than life', whilst others have lived for many years 'merging into the background'. Some people have dominant personalities and others are more passive. Some people are by nature extrovert and others are by nature introvert. In recent years there has been a considerable amount of work done exploring the nature of people's personalities (see for instance Goldsmith and Wharton 1993). When people become ill, they bring their personalities with them into the experience of their illness. It is therefore of crucial importance that we understand, as well as we are able, just what sort of a person we are relating to. What the underlying traits and characteristics likely to be? No one type of person is 'better' than another, but they are different, and it is helpful if we can begin to see how their illness overlays and finds expression in their basic personality. It may be that some personality profiles are able to adjust and accept the experience of dementia more easily than others; we just do not know enough about this area at the moment.

Not only are the personalities different, so too are the illnesses which are commonly lumped together under the heading of 'dementia'. Alzheimer's disease is the most prevalent, followed by multi-infarct dementia (arterio-sclerotic or vascular dementia). Other illnesses can also bring dementia: Parkinson's disease, Lewy body disease, Korsakoff's syndrome, Huntington's chorea, Creutzfeldt-Jakob (C-J) disease, or those related to the AIDS virus. There is a tendency for people to talk in a general way about Alzheimer's disease, without recognising that it is a quite specific disease. Whilst some people talk about 'dementia' as though that were a specific disease rather than being a generic name, or more precisely a 'syndrome' – which means that it is a characteristic pattern of clinical features which can be caused by one or more of a number of specific illnesses. Whilst there are general signs and symptoms which, when put together we can call 'dementia', each illness has its own specific pattern and characteristics.

We are increasingly becoming aware of the view that the biomedical understanding of these illnesses is intimately linked to the psychosocial condition of each person, so that what emerges is a quite distinct and unique person, patient or client. As Mills and Chapman (1992) observe:

> Irreversible dementia therefore, is not merely a disease caused by biological changes in the brain. It is an illness which has psychological and social processes which give good reason to believe that social and

psychological factors influence symptom formation and the course of dementia. (p.27)

As a professor in the health care of the elderly commented:

> Different people are indeed affected in different ways, and different dementing illnesses affect people in different ways. Those that particularly alter personality, such as chronic degenerative disorders like Alzheimer's disease often make the biggest differences and cause greatest difficulty for carers, whereas others, for example some cases of vascular dementia do not present in this way. On the other hand, damage to certain parts of the brain in vascular dementia can lead to major behavioural changes. It is important to carefully profile an individual subject and then devise a treatment programme that is specific for that individual. It must also take into account the personality of the carer.

A consultant physician in geriatric medicine called for much more thorough testing so that the precise nature of the illness might better be diagnosed:

> the label of dementia is of little actual use. Attempts to define the nature of chronic organic brain syndromes are vital. Furthermore, screening, psychological and if necessary full psychological assessment of higher cognitive functions would enable the identification of specific deficits and thus ways to cope with them. This has a resource implication in terms of clinical psychology availability, but also a training and educational issue for carers (formal and informal) and health professionals.

What we have therefore are different types of personality which might be affected by different illnesses. Another variant of growing importance is that of the age of the person with dementia. As diagnostic techniques improve, it is likely that more people will be diagnosed at an earlier age and the pressure for services to be more age-related will grow. Many people wrote in commenting on the fact that we should not assume that people in their fifties or sixties necessarily have a lot in common with people in their eighties and nineties, and yet a great many of our facilities and services place them all together.

The majority of people with dementia are still elderly though, and therefore are more likely to have additional illnesses or disabilities. Few people seem to suffer from dementia alone and there are invariably additional factors which have to be taken into consideration: failing eyesight or hearing, restricted mobility, and psychosocial conditions such as loneliness, bereavement and depression. Many people wrote in saying that failure to provide adequate spectacles, dentures or hearing aids made the whole process of communicating with people with dementia that much more difficult.

Added to all these factors must be an acknowledgement that the same person can vary a great deal in how they react and behave, according to a different set of variables. The time of day, before or after meals, before or after they are about to receive a service (for example, attendance at a day care centre), can all make a difference. Similarly, they may react differently according to whether they are within their own homes or in some other setting, and whether they are surrounded by people whom they know or whether there are people around whom they cannot identify. These many different situations and contexts can yield quite different information. There can also be differences depending upon the consistency of approach and continuity of carers. What is quite obvious, therefore, is that there needs to be a considerable investment of time and skills in order to understand where the person is at this moment, and where they are coming from, and in order to facilitate a communicative process.

The overwhelming number of replies on this topic referred to the need for individualised care plans, and the need for respecting the person and making them the centre of whatever was being decided. A few people wrote in to say that people *were* being treated differently, but not in the way that I was hoping to hear. An inspector wrote:

> there is a major difference in attitude in staff treatment of different people. Those who are 'happy and quiet', often provoking a benign paternalism from staff. Those with challenging behaviours, however, being treated as being naughty or 'doing it on purpose'.

Dementia Care Mapping, which an increasing number of establishments are now using in order to establish an indicator of well-being, was cited as illustrating how it is possible to demonstrate that people are treated in different ways irrespective of their actual needs. A project worker commented:

> Sadly, different people are treated very differently. The further into dementia that people sink, the less good will be their experience of care. My Dementia Care Mapping project bears this out. People's Individual Care Scores reflect their ability levels; the more able the person, the better the score; the more disabled the person, the lower the score. I think services could be far more 'user-sensitive' if we adopted the hospice model of having a team of about five staff responsible between them for any given individual. This would mean

that the person would always and only be cared for by one of her team – and the team would have to organise their leave etc. between them. This way, an improved continuity of care would result.

An even more contentious point was made by a ward manager:

> I have now worked in four Health Authorities/Trusts and the social divide is to me the most obvious inequality affecting care. I do not wish to get political, but I feel the Community Care Act is heavily slanted against the lower classes and the medical model employed by many consultants leads to a favourable response to those better educated and able to express their needs more eloquently. Provision of private care is obviously better the more finance is available, giving a clear advantage to the rich over those requiring social service funding.

If we are to see the person with dementia as a 'whole person', if we are to respect and honour the person despite their cognitive impairment, then it is important that we build up as full a picture of them as possible. This includes the social and relationship aspects as well as the biomedical, as Kitwood (1990a) reminds us:

> human beings are far more deeply affected by the social psychology that surrounds them than is commonly recognised. In particular, the maintenance of self-esteem is essential for good learning, efficacy and constructive relationships with others. Conversely, when self-esteem is lacking or damaged, a person is disastrously incapacitated in many ways, and easily falls into a cycle of discouragement and failure…each aspect of the malignant social psychology is, in some way, damaging to self-esteem, and tends to diminish personhood; that is why it merits the epithet 'malignant'…remarkably, the greater part of medical science research on dementia seems to overlook this altogether. (p.181)

There is an urgent need to retain a biographical perspective on people with dementia and to combine this with a sense of their personal value as people. This is something that I shall return to in Chapter 8.

Reflecting on the responses

From the 200 plus comments that I received on this issue, I was interested to note that there was an overwhelming desire to stress the importance of viewing the person as an individual. On the other hand, there also seemed to be an underlying tension between the ideal of responding to people with dementia as individuals and the constraints placed upon so many people working in the field by limited time and resources. What they write about might be called, as someone described it – a 'dream service', meaning the sort of service that they really hoped to provide but which, in reality, they knew only too well they were failing to deliver. They were very aware of the problems they had in delivering such a service. One social worker wrote:

> all services should be focused on the individual – individual care plans are an ideal way of doing this and we have introduced them into our residential homes *and are about to do so* into our Home Care Service. [my italics]

What we have here is a recognition of the 'dream service' or 'ideal service' and a partial response to it. Whilst many people wrote about the need for a service which was specifically tailored to meet the needs of younger people with dementia, not a single response detailed how they had brought such a service into being. The ideal or dream service was put forward with conviction, but the reality of much that was being provided seemed to challenge what was being said. The problem with describing it as a dream service is that dreams are never realised, whilst what we are wanting is a service which matches the very best that we can hope to achieve – a service which *is* capable of being delivered, given the right circumstances and will.

One consultant focused on the low status of the work undertaken in caring for people with dementia and highlighted managerial decisions to amalgamate differing dementia wards to create larger groups of people with the underlying purpose, one assumes, of saving money. This has the effect of producing residential services which run counter to the dream service which so many people talk about. The demoralisation that such an event caused amongst staff, and the subsequent need to systematise routines to cater for larger numbers is an ever present reality in much dementia care, and yet few respondents grappled with the situation as it now is, preferring to set out their ideals for what the service might be.

The responses from carers seemed to have a greater immediacy about them and they repeatedly described situations in which there obviously was a failure to provide high standard individualised care, and they conveyed a deep sense of longing for it.

> The other people in the centre my father attends are very different to him and communicate differently...while he is extremely placid and friendly, others communicate in an aggressive manner, or don't speak; others weep all day.

Whilst another carer commented that:

> I have seen docile people suffer terrible bruising, broken limbs and
> lacerations from those more aggressive…there needs to be separation
> between these groups because the docile do nothing to protect
> themselves, even when falling, for example. The more violent should
> be accommodated separately. The younger sufferers should also be
> accommodated separately from the elderly to combat depression.
> There is need for continuity in all aspects of caring.

These carers obviously want an individualised, needs-led, segregated service
for their relatives, but they are not receiving it. They see people inappropriately placed and lumped together with others on the basis of the diagnosis
of dementia, and who knows what distress is being endured by the relatives
and their carers?

Grouping people together

Quite a number of people wrote in describing problems they had when
people were grouped together merely because they had a diagnosis of
dementia. The principal ways in which people are grouped together is in
all-age groups, and in groups which bring together people with differing
degrees of impairment. One charge nurse in an elderly mentally infirm unit
described this as being 'very disrespectful' and said that in her view it
undermined people's individuality. It needs to be remembered that this is the
norm in dementia care. One person wrote in saying that

> this probably throws up the old discussion around integration versus
> segregation. At which point do people need access to specialist
> services as opposed to generic services? And, to a lesser extent, it raises
> the issue of whether we need to have diagnosis of dementia at all if it
> is likely to result in people being treated with less respect for
> individuality.

The head of an occupational therapy unit confessed to 'only having experience of "lumping people together"', and a human resources development
manager said 'I do not personally have sufficient experience of treating
people in different ways'. What seemed to emerge from the replies to my
consultative document was a growing awareness of the need for individualised care plans, the importance of treating each person with respect, and yet
the knowledge that this is not always the case and the acknowledgment that

there would be cost implications if a satisfactory service were to be provided as a matter of course.

Specialised and flexible services

Service provision needs to be as flexible and innovative as possible. Time and time again people wrote in expressing a desire for greater flexibility. A typical comment was:

> We need flexibility in how services are provided: a variety of care settings and packages rather than the usual result of placing people with dementia into spaces in existing care.

It is the old problem of do we allocate available services to people who need them, or do we provide the services which they need? That is, is service delivery dictated by supply or by demand? In one sense it is the chicken and egg issue all over again, and yet there is sufficient truth in the view that we need greater flexibility for us to need to take a serious look again at just what is being provided, when, where and for whom. There are too many examples of people in residential establishments having only sparse snacks in the evening because the staff have gone home, or of people spending inordinate amounts of time in minibuses being ferried around on pick-up trips, or of services not being available at the times which would be most convenient. The example of evening day-care which is provided in Cowdenbeath (Carr 1995) could be replicated in many other places, but it remains a fairly rare example. There is also still little evidence of people being involved in their own care planning.

One person, a clinical neuropsychologist, commented on the need for services to be available which were more specifically tailored for ethnic minorities:

> there are very few services, if any, for people from different ethnic minority groups. It would be exciting to organise facilities which took into account ethnic and religious backgrounds. Day care in a mosque, special services in church or temple, counselling from a rabbi, etc...

Speakers at a workshop at the 1994 Alzheimer's Disease International Conference in Edinburgh told of a scheme in Pennsylvania in which local black churches were providing specialist care for a group of people who had consistently failed to be supported by mainstream services. The service providers had gone out of their way to provide care in a format and in a context which would be acceptable to a population which was inherently suspicious of, and apprehensive about, the majority community.

The deputy manager of a home for older people wrote about what flexibility meant in that context:

> The experience of dementia is different for everyone and approaches have to be individualised. This was particularly evident when I was asked to work in the community. You can find two people with similar degrees of dementia – one would become anxious, upset, timid and frightened, and the other could become over-confident, reassured, dismissive of care. Some workers would have a standard residential care option for both clients. I tended to tolerate higher levels of risk. The first person would probably be reassured by being surrounded by people in residential care and this could be an appropriate course of action. The second would probably feel she had been removed against her will and feel imprisoned. This would be acted out in different behaviour. For the sake of psychological health I do feel that we need to take risks. Clearly there has to be a point when a person with dementia cannot live in the community, and allowing them to live in their own excrement, fry their knickers under the grill and keep their shoes in the fridge is far from empowering. Nevertheless, I feel that there needs to be a loose and creative response which leaves the person with dementia feeling that they have some control over what is happening to them.

Some interesting work is being done in small group work and in small living units. A customer services manager writes that ideally people should live in small units if they are no longer able to live in their own home:

> this would prevent people in different stages of dementia being lumped together. For example, some people still have social skills and are able to eat and drink and talk, whereas others haven't. If people are together in small groups, it is essential to undertake reassessments every three months to ensure that they are still appropriately placed.

An inspector stressed the importance of individual care plans which genuinely strive to identify people's likes, dislikes, previous lifestyles, interests and behaviour. He emphasised that individual care plans are central to good practice and that these are valid in both residential and non-residential settings, but 'they are expensive in staff time'. Someone who did work almost entirely on a one-to-one basis said 'I am constantly adapting to the variety of personalities I encounter. Such flexibility is essential if progress in getting to know sufferers as persons is to be made'. As one of them said to him, 'I didn't know if you would understand, with you living on the other side'.

Families also are different

It is perhaps worth mentioning that just as the people with dementia are unique beings, each with their own personality and each needing to be understood and valued, so too carers and families are different, and they have different ways of coping. One clinical psychologist commented:

> we were thinking of working out the parameters involved in the way different families cope with admission to long-term care because of dementia. In first discussions we thought relevant variables are the relationship of the resident to the relative, pre-existing family relationships and the way the admission has been handled by the services supporting the family. How to help the family means being clear about where they are with all this. There can be no assumptions about what kind of support particular individuals and families need.

The need for sustained training

Coping with people on an individual basis is not always easy and being prepared to accept the differences of personality as well as the different experiences of the illness can be a demanding task for staff. Having the imagination and the ability to prepare individual and flexible care plans does not come easy, and there is often the temptation to impose routines which are convenient for the service rather than adapt the service to the needs of the individual. Being as committed to the difficult and the noisy person as you are to the pleasant and the amenable person demands considerable skill and determination. There is the need for those who are working face to face with the person with dementia, to know that they have the support of their superiors in providing a service which is flexible and tailored to meet individual need. This is not always easy to provide in situations where resources are limited, but as one service manager reflected:

> the person-centred approach advocated by Tom Kitwood allows for differences between individuals when practised in a residential setting. Additional time is necessary for the preparation of staff, but client satisfaction with the approach eventually makes caring easier and infinitely more satisfying.

A development nurse in dementia services set out the scope of the problem.

> Approachable, formal and informal teaching sessions should be aimed to all healthcare professionals working in adult health. During the course of my frequent teaching sessions I am amazed at how little people understand about dementia, and how often it is used as an umbrella term for all manner of conditions. Staff are always responsive and usually astounded when they realise the true nature of the problem. Sensitively conducted education programmes can usually uncover a mine of suppositions and misunderstandings. 'Individualised care' is a term that is often bandied about. Specialists working in the field have a responsibility to pass on their knowledge and experience to empower staff to carry this out.

Finally, a clinical services manager summed up what she thought all this entailed:

> It is important for all staff to understand the physiological and pathological process of the disease. The more knowledge and understanding staff have of the illness the more the patient will benefit in terms of experience and skill. Each person with dementia is an individual with their own set of circumstances and needs and it is important to obtain full detailed history from the person and the carers. Following the initial assessment a package of care tailored to the individual can be discussed within a multidisciplinary team that includes the person with dementia and carers.

> As the illness progresses there are different stages of dependency which have to be dealt with as they arise. If the person with dementia remains at home, consideration has to be given to the needs of the carer. The main aspect of service providers has to be a flexible approach that can respond to unexpected situations quickly and efficiently. The main aim should be to maintain the person in their own home for as long as it is feasible, practical and safe to do so. A provider service should have the following available:

> - A multidisciplinary mental health team that includes medical and nursing staff, social worker, psychologist and occupational therapist.
> - A community psychiatric nurse, who plays a key role in supporting people with dementia and their carers in the community.
> - A well planned package of relief admissions.

- Provision of day care, in either a day hospital or a voluntary day centre.
- Close liaison with social services to refer on to – home care…meals on wheels…residential or nursing home.

Conclusions

If we are serious in our endeavours to hear the voices of people with dementia, then we have to recognise that no two people are the same, and that each person will present us with quite specific and unique challenges. Not only will their basic personality be different from that of others, but also their network of relationships, their own history and experiences, the state of their general health and the specific situation regarding their dementing illness. All these factors have to be taken into consideration as we draw up a plan of care for them, and with them. What 'works' with one person will not necessarily work with another. Staff need training to develop special skills and also to enlarge their general understanding of the pattern of the illnesses which produce dementia. There is always going to be potential tension between working with individuals at depth and working within the constraints of limited resources, but at least let us be honest about where the problems lie. The major problem may not necessarily be the inability of the person with dementia to communicate, but our inability to afford them the appropriate amount of time and the individualised attention that they need at this stage of their illness.

CHAPTER 5

Communication is Possible

This is a crucial chapter. We have to answer the basic question as to whether we actually believe that it is possible to communicate – or not. If we believe that it is possible, then this will radically alter the ways in which we endeavour to overcome the obstacles and explore the possibilities.

Two long-term processes of communication are described, together with a daughter's approach to her mother's communicative difficulties.

Some of the technical difficulties are mentioned, together with the exploration of some strategies for facilitating better communication. Specific problems for people from other cultures are noted.

When I was a child, I wondered if Grandma was born old. I could not imagine her laughing, teasing, or being anyone's friend. My conception of her was of an old woman who spoke broken English and bound vinegar-soaked cabbage leaves around her head. I could not understand my mother's devotion to her because she wreaked such havoc on our family. There were countless times she stood outside our back door and screamed untrue verbal abuse at my mother. So many nights were spent in vigils while Grandma prowled her house hiding things she could not find the next morning. How did my mother balance family and career while meeting the constant demands of caring for Grandma? Why did she refuse other family members' solution of 'putting Grandma away' when the alternative was her own physical and mental distress?... Little did I realise that these experiences of a grammar-school child would generate my philosophy that communication with elderly individuals with dementia is important...verbal and nonverbal communication links us to the essence of a person's humanity. Each time we communicate with the elderly demented we are called upon to use all of our adaptive and creative skills...many times it seemed easier to avoid talking than trying to understand and respond to the demented individual...

Perhaps after reading this you will say 'this is too much: there really isn't anything that can be done'. Dementia will seem like an insurmountable slope that slides back with every step of progress. Let us as individuals and as a profession be defined not by the goals we have accomplished but by the challenges that we try to meet. (Lubinski 1991a, p.xi)

These words are taken from the Preface of a large book on the subject of dementia and communication. Rosemary Lubinski does not minimise the difficulty of the task, but she is quite sure that communication is possible. The questions to be asked are:

- is it possible with all people?
- what degree of communication are we talking about?
- what forms might this communication take?
- and are there any strategies or techniques which can help in the communicative process?

My own project was to explore the extent to which people with dementia might have their voices heard when considering the services that they were receiving. The consultative document that I sent out invited comment from people working in the field on ten key areas, the first of which was that *communication with people with dementia is possible*, and my assertion was that:

It is possible, but it can be a difficult and slow process, requiring time, patience, skill and commitment. If communication is possible, then it must be possible to communicate about services, and for the majority of people with dementia it must be possible for them to communicate their satisfaction (or dissatisfaction) with the services provided. Not to pursue this task of eliciting such views is tantamount to saying either that they are unable to communicate or that their views are irrelevant to service providers.

The vast majority of the replies were in general agreement with the statement, some of them enthusiastically supportive, but there were several words of caution from others. A psychiatrist wrote 'in my experience, judgment is one of the first cognitive functions lost in many demented patients. I think a committed "ideological" approach to eliciting patients' views on services would be unlikely to lie in their interest and would, in fact, be largely a waste of time and effort'. A ward manager wrote in saying:

Communication with people with dementia is possible, though I do not necessarily accept that you can make a clear link between this and identifying service provision. In my experience, by the time dementia is diagnosed there is an associated lack of insight into their condition, leading them to make unrealistic demands on service provision.

A senior social worker echoed this sense of people being 'unrealistic in what they communicate'. On the other hand a director of quality replied saying:

We have often received feedback from people with dementia, as well as their relatives, which have helped us in service developments in the past. We have also recently upbraided our main purchaser for consulting only with carers and have put them in touch with people in earlier stages of dementia who were interviewed. This contributed significantly to the strategic direction part of their purchasing intentions.

Obviously one of the important factors is the severity of a person's illness and quite a number of people wrote in complaining that once the label of 'dementia' was given to someone, a great many people assumed that they had nothing to contribute and that their views or expressions were almost certain to be distorted and unintelligible. As one officer in charge of a residential home observed:

in my experience most people tend to enter into a one-way communication system with people with dementia. People tend to speak to the client and not wait for a response, or at best, give the response for the person. When questioned about this practice people tend often to say that they know what the person wants. I have found the only way to communicate is on a one-to-one basis and devote as much time as possible to the client.

A charge nurse in an Elderly Mentally Infirm (EMI) acute assessment ward was in no doubt as to the reality of the problem:

Many service providers expect people with dementia *not* to have a voice or be able to express an opinion. The whole culture is in need of change. The general public seem to associate the term 'dementia' with a vegetative state...in my opinion it is a very demeaning and derogatory name for what is a very complex and individualised process. It does seem that as soon as a diagnosis of this nature is made then in many cases individuals are expected to conform to a pattern of 'dementia type behaviour' thus superseding any individuality he or

she may have. It takes a lot of time to get to know a person well –
extra time and effort must be put aside in order to get to know
someone who has changed with the aging process and may have
become ill or forgetful.

Comments such as this, and many others, reinforce what Smithers (1977)
found in her study of a nursing home. She wrote that 'in coming to be viewed
as senile, patients are judged incapable of functioning rationally and assume
a less than human aspect'. Also, she claimed, such patients are freed from the
expectations made of more rational patients and therefore tend to take on
the status of a non-person.

What seems to emerge is an overwhelming conviction that it is possible
to communicate with people with dementia, but that it takes time and skill.
If we are not prepared to change our own attitudes and approach then we
may well find the communicative process well nigh impossible, but if we
regard it as a challenge to be overcome, then the evidence suggests that
communication is possible far longer than is normally expected.

Gemma Jones (1992) comments that the rules for communicating with
normal healthy people have to be completely altered when working with a
person with Alzheimer's disease.

> The rules for normal communication demand a fairly equal exchange
> between two communicating parties; in working with people with
> dementia the exchange cannot be equal and a care-giver must make a
> decision to provide extra energy and input into the communication if
> it is to be a meaningful one. (p.77)

To illustrate that communication *is* possible, even in quite advanced stages,
I want to comment upon two longitudinal studies which I found to be of
particular interest. This chapter is primarily concerned with verbal communication; there are of course other forms of communication and these will
be looked at in greater detail later.

Two conversations over time

Valerie Sinason (1992) is a psychotherapist who spends much of her time in
practice with people who have considerable mental or physical disabilities,
or both. One such person was Edward Johnson, an academic whom she
visited on an almost weekly basis for a year; she then wrote up her reflections
on that process. She begins by considering the experience of loss. Loss is
something which we all have to cope with, from the moment we are born,
and every new phase of our living involves loss. Underlying all these

experiences is an awareness of our own mortality. She comments that a person born with only one hand is still born with 'a concept of two hands just as a child without a father still has an image of a father'. 'A child or adult without a fully functioning brain lives with the shadow of the missing part' (p.88).

> ...any change that goes beyond what is realistically expected and emotionally prepared for attacks our central belief in ourselves as autonomous beings. With the advent of a sudden pain, illness, injury that was not self-afflicted, we face yet again our own mortality.
>
> With Alzheimer's disease, there is not only a physical impact, there is a measurable mental deterioration too. From knowing, possessing knowledge, words, thoughts, there is a downward path to not knowing. It means returning back to the first chaos of infancy when not an infant and having possessed knowledge at its fullest and finest. The difference between someone at the start of Alzheimer's disease and someone near the end is as large as the difference between someone who is normal and someone who is profoundly handicapped. The total continuum is experienced in the mind and heart of a single being. (p.89)

Edward Johnson was a university teacher at the height of his profession, 'he prided himself on the breadth and depth of his academic scholarship and travelled the globe to share it. Now even a few steps and he is lost'. He was referred to her by the GP, who was worried about the devastating emotional and cognitive impact of his condition. There then followed a year of meetings in which they were able to explore his self-understanding and his emotional and intellectual reactions to his illness. Eventually they reached a stage when he said 'I do not want to be rude, but I do not want to think any more', and they closed their sessions. This chapter in Sinason's book is a profoundly moving observation of, and insight into, the slow deterioration of a mind and the problems of communicating. It is also a helpful model for understanding how to relate and communicate. Few of us will have her psychotherapeutic skills, but it is helpful to realise that people with those skills also experience similar sorts of confusion and helplessness as we sometimes do ourselves when endeavouring to engage in meaningful conversation with a person with dementia. I found helpful her observation that it is essential (for therapists – but also, presumably for others as well) to be able to bear 'not knowing what they do not know, and being honest about it'. This resonates with what Kitwood has said about being confronted with our own vulnerability when we are engaged in this sort of dialogue.

The second extended conversation with someone who has Alzheimer's disease is a more technical book, an interactional sociolinguistic study by Heidi Ehernberger Hamilton (1994). This is an account of how an elderly woman's communicative abilities and disabilities changed over a four and a half year period. It looks at how they are influenced by the role of the author, as she both initiates and responds to conversations. In the introduction to the book Hamilton says

> I hope the reader will come to know a person with wishes, needs, and intentions, who laughs, gets embarrassed, expresses happiness, confidence and confusion, and shows love and concern for others – an individual who is both hindered and helped by her conversational partner to success in interaction. Elsie's language reflects the mental disability of Alzheimer's disease and holds in it countless secrets regarding her abilities and disabilities. (p.1)

When this study began, in 1981, Elsie 'issued requests, expressed wishes, asked for information and clarification, expressed concern for others, provided excuses for her unexpected behaviour and refused offers – all by use of linguistic means' (p.148). When the period of observation and interaction came to a close, four and a half years later, she 'not once initiated an exchange verbally, but only responded to my utterances...without using words' (p.148). Hamilton suggests that Elsie passes through four stages. Stage one is active, confused and aware; stage two is active, confused and unaware, stage three is less active, confused and unaware, and finally she describes stage four as passive – but even here she is still able to 'request repetition of her conversational partner's utterance, to take conversational turns appropriately, and to indicate that she recognizes personally important topics' (p.159) – doing this by a variety of sounds which Hamilton is able to interpret.

What both these studies show is that if the will is there and if the person has relevant skills, then it is possible to converse with people with dementia through to a very late stage in the illness. It is not acceptable at an early stage, nor even at a later stage for that matter, to write off a person's ability to communicate just because we find it difficult to comprehend what they are trying to convey to us. If there is a problem in understanding then the responsibility lies with us to ensure that we are doing everything possible to facilitate communication.

Some technical reflections
Christine De Luca, who wrote the poem in the previous chapter about the Church of Scotland minister, wrote another one following a later visit.

You look different today
despite the smile.
Is it the lack of tie
or the poor shave?

Bits of sentences collapse
between brain and mouth:
a computer file struck
by a virus. Gaps which dangle
between nouns are too big
for leaps of inference;
there is anxiety
in both words and pauses:
it is tempting to smooth
their edges with inconsequentials.
Having lost the past and future
it seems that you are pure being;
that you have made each instant
your stillest dwelling.

Yet you can smile that smile forever you
to take us back, and lead us on:
that simplest of complexities
remains.   (De Luca unpublished)

Sandra Walker, writing in 1988, commented on how little information was really known about the speech of people with dementia. She commented that until the late seventies there was little scientific data on the language of dementia, and 'as with any developing art, a lack of universality of terms, definitions and populations' frequently complicates the data that is available. She said that a lack of information through ignorance of the extent of the problem, and a paucity of scientific data on all aspects of the disease, especially on the linguistic features, has created a complex and fragmented database. There had also been little evaluation or research done specifically on communication, and there had been virtually no evaluation of strategies or cost effectiveness.

In 1991 Virginia Lee undertook a literature review on Alzheimer's disease and language issues and she admitted that the cognitive changes which occur in individuals with dementia are not clearly or completely understood, but their effects on language and on the ability of people to communicate and interact appropriately with others are very considerable indeed. In a study in 1982 communication difficulties were found to be the sixth most common problem causing stress to carers; the other five, which were thought to be more stressful, were memory disturbances, catastrophic reactions, demanding and critical behaviour, night waking and hiding things. The ability to communicate, both verbally and nonverbally, is a critical component of effective caring for people with dementia, and a breakdown in communication can be at best irritating and at worst overwhelming for those who are doing the caring.

It is recognised that problems in communication, when added to other problematic behaviours, can easily lead to frustration, anger and the desire to ignore the person and, of course, this is precisely what happens in so many situations. We are slowly building up resource material which can help people in the process of communication – gaining eye contact, using simple sentence constructions, giving one-step instructions, minimising distractions and so forth, and these will be described later, but what we know much less about are the actual changes in language that occur with dementia and how different dementing illnesses may produce different patterns of speech deterioration.

We know something of the pattern of breakdown of language in Alzheimer's disease. The first change that occurs is in tasks such as naming – in that aspect of language which is concerned with the meaning of words (semantic system). Then follows a process of deviation and simplification of grammar (syntax), and then the disordered use of sounds (phonetic breakdown) (see Stevens *et al.* 1992). Griffiths (1991) comments that there is probably language disturbance at all stages in Alzheimer's disease, and studies show how these develop as the disease progresses. In the early stages of the disease speech is often described as being fluent, circuitous, empty and vague, with incomplete utterances. Word-finding problems become apparent in conversation, and the inability to name things becomes noticeable. As the disease progresses speech becomes increasingly repetitive, with less attention paid to conversational rules, and it appears to be increasingly egocentric. This may be followed by mutism. Interestingly, it appears that the ability to read aloud often remains, to a relatively late stage, although comprehension of what is read may have long since been eroded.

We know much less about how language changes occur in people who do not have English as their first language. If a person's second language is English, and is already that much more fragile, then considerable caution will be needed when analysing the results of language testing and, of course, general communication will be that much more difficult. This will become an increasing problem as an immigrant population from non-English speaking countries grows older. We also know less about how speech is affected by forms of dementia other than Alzheimer's disease, because even less research has been done in those areas.

Some variable factors

The ability of people to communicate will vary from person to person and will be influenced by a number of factors. The principal factor is the stage that the disease has reached. In almost all cases, communicative ability deteriorates the more advanced the illness, although we must take care not to compare one person's ability with another's and draw conclusions about the relative stages of their illness, because in some people language will go fairly quickly and with others its loss may be slower and deterioration becomes more marked in other facets of their life.

One clinical psychologist wrote in saying:

> The whole issue of communication seems to me to be very complex indeed, involving at least two people and content, which interact with each other in a variety of ways. To ask if *A* can communicate strikes me as being only part of the question which should in fact be *Can A communicate with B about X?* There is no likelihood of significant communication unless a trusting relationship already exists...I believe that if trust is there, the person will find some way of communicating what needs to be communicated.

A consultant physician in elderly medicine, whilst agreeing that communication with people with dementia in general terms was possible, felt that it was too broad a generalisation. He wrote in saying

> it depends upon the extent of the disease and the higher cognitive functions involved. For example, for patients with gross dysphasia, meaningful spoken or written communication is not necessarily possible. For those with severe Alzheimer's disease I suspect that although some degree of communication is possible, meaningful comment about their satisfaction with services is not actually possible in any direct manner. If you are not aware of your environment then you are not in a position to directly comment upon it. I would, however, fully accept that immediate physical responses to environmental stimuli may give some overall feeling about a person's reaction, but this is not necessarily the same thing as satisfaction.

He went on to suggest that asking people to choose their menus a week in advance – thus in theory extending their choice – was, in fact, giving them less choice than offering them a choice of two alternative meals, both of which they could see, at any mealtime.

Other variable factors which will be discussed later will be the time of day, the location, the person with whom communication is taking place, and the number of external distractions such as noise, or people moving about. It is quite clear that someone who is apparently unable to communicate much in one situation, at another time and in another place, might be quite lucid. And of course, the reverse is also true, and a person who seems to be able to hold their own quite well may, in a different situation, be apparently quite unable to understand what is being said or what is happening. To distinguish these different states demands time, patience and skill on the part of the person giving care or attempting to communicate.

Strategies for communication

Gemma Jones (1992) observes that many residents in nursing and residential homes can be thought of as having been sentenced to solitary confinement without a trial. She says that the only chance that they have of communicating and sharing fragments of their normal lives is through the efforts of those staff members and carers who do not pass judgment on their behaviour, and who try to remove as many of the barriers to communication as possible. If a person does not hear their name spoken several times a day and if they are not encouraged to use their speech, however inadequate it might be, and if they are not stimulated to express themselves in whatever ways that they are able to, then 'by how much and how quickly are they deteriorating unnecessarily?'

Before looking at specific techniques, it is worth mentioning a few general 'ground rules'. These are concerned with the attitude of mind that we bring to the process of communication. We may have all manner of techniques and skills, but if we lack these basic ingredients, then our attempts to communicate will prove far more difficult that if we had few techniques but were rich in these basics. Possibly the most important of all is the ability to listen. Second to that comes the ability to accept the person as they are and to accept the possibilities of communication, and once we can accept these, then we are on the way to understanding – however long it may take us.

Lam and Beech (1994, section 2) quote Kitwood as suggesting that 'the best thing is to treat everything (that the person with dementia) says, however jumbled and fantastic it may seem to be, as an attempt to tell us something'. He suggests that it is rather like us being interpreters of a foreign language and there are as many differences within dementia as there are different foreign languages. The important thing is that we do not allow ourselves to become all hung up on the literal meaning of words, rather we need to look for the hidden meaning that lies behind the words. We need to get a 'feel' for the sense that is behind them, we need to 'slow down our thought processes, to become inwardly quiet, and to have a kind of poetic awareness'. It is more an art than a science. We need to look for metaphor and illusion rather than 'pursuing meaning with a relentless kind of tunnel vision'. In the same article, Lam and Beech quote Naomi Feil, and suggest that, when in the role of 'validating caregiver', we need to release any feelings of anger or frustration that we might harbour, and we need to pay attention to the form of our words, our tone, our posture and the nature of our eye contact. She also recommends that we use questions beginning with *when, where* and *who,* rather than those beginning with *why.*

Tom Kitwood (1993) paints a graphic picture of the process of communication. If successful communication is to take place then the carer, the person without dementia, must play a rather different role from that taken in everyday communication. He or she must learn some of the skills more associated with the counsellor. The more severe a person's dementia is, then the greater will be the need for the other person to have these communicative skills. Kitwood uses the image of tennis. The carer is rather like the experienced tennis coach who is able to keep a rally going with the less experienced person on the other side of the net. Wherever that person plays the ball the coach seems able to reach it and return it. But he returns it in such a way as to keep the rally going. He does not return it in order to score a point or win the match, but rather he returns the ball so that the other player is able to reach it and, with encouragement, is able to play it back over the net again. Similarly with our communication with a person with dementia, it is possible to learn techniques which 'keep open' the conversation and which allow the person with dementia to respond.[1]

What follows here is a compilation of many of the ideas that different people have suggested, either in their written comments to me or in the literature that is currently available. It is not intended to cover every aspect of communication, and no doubt each of the points could be subdivided, and others could be added. However, it is a useful 'rough and ready guide' to use in the process of communication.

---

1   For those wanting more detailed information on communication *Coping with Communication Challenges in Alzheimer's Disease* (1993) by Marie T Rau is excellent, and easy to read and understand. She has also contributed a chapter to the Rosemary Lubinski (1991a) book referred to earlier.

◦ Make sure that the environment is conducive for communication. The noise of the radio or television should not be competing with your voice. People should not be hurrying by or engaged in noisy activities in the same room.

◦ Ensure that you yourself are calm and do not appear to be flustered or under time pressures. You will need to be able to give the person your full attention – this can be tiring, and you will be unlikely to be able to do it well if your mind is on something else at the same time. Try to ensure that your facial expression and body posture are reassuring and relaxed.

◦ Approach them within their line of vision, and try not to surprise or startle them. Identify yourself, by introducing yourself by name, even if you are well known. Also, if appropriate, use their name as well. Establish eye contact, and if possible speak to them from the same level.

◦ Use touch to reinforce your presence and what you are saying – but establish first whether this is appropriate. Do not force touch onto someone who does not want it.

◦ Speak simply, and slowly, but do not 'speak down' to the person. Always endeavour to maintain their dignity.

◦ Allow time for them to understand what you are saying. Remember that even with moderate dementia it can take five times longer to process information than it takes for an elderly person without the illness. Make sure that they understand before you move the conversation on.

◦ Be a good listener. Communication is a two-way process and you need to be alert to pick up clues and prompts. Do not be afraid of long pauses, and do not jump in and complete sentences for the person whilst they are in the process of formulating them. Listen for what they are saying 'behind the words'. Remember that elderly people often speak metaphorically, and this is particularly so with dementia.

◦ Do not assume that they do not understand just because they have not responded straight away. They may not have understood, but on the other hand, they may be only too aware of what you are saying but either cannot, or do not want to respond.

◦ Use short sentences and do not carry double messages in them. 'Would you like to have a cup of tea and then go for a walk?' should be divided up into two distinct sentences, and the first one dealt with before the second is introduced.

- ○ If at all possible, illustrate what you are saying – use photographs when talking about someone, show them the cardigan if you are asking if they want to put it on, and use your hands and body language to support what you are wanting to communicate. Make sure that your illustrations match your words – don't show a photograph of A and talk about B!

- ○ Even if their thought process or their use of words gets mixed up, you may still be able to follow what they are trying to say. Do not feel that you have to correct their mistakes, and do not laugh at their attempts, even when they have totally misunderstood you or responded inappropriately.

- ○ Be complimentary if it is appropriate – but in an adult manner. It may be taking a great effort to converse with you, and show your pleasure when they succeed.

- ○ Do not be embarrassed by a display of emotion, whether it is tearful or one of anger. If it is something that needs to come out, then do not attempt to avoid it. You may be helping them a great deal by providing a context and enabling a process which helps them to express their innermost feelings or anxieties.

Communication is not always easy, and we all need encouragement if we are to persevere. It may be more important to 'stick in there' when the response is minimal or non-existent than when there is a certain ease and rapport building up. If those people who know that communication is important feel that they don't have enough time or energy for it, then those who are less aware of its value are all the more likely to give in earlier, and one more person is destined to spend yet more time locked up in their own world.

What I do not recommend is following the advice from a Japanese writer on dementia (Takahiro 1991). Amidst his rules for better nursing care come these gems: 'How important it is to understand the world of the elderly. That is a fundamental rule when talking to them. Pretend that you are acting so that you don't have a guilty conscience even if you have lied to them…the aged should be treated as human beings, *or as patients*, but not as a nuisance…sometimes it is necessary to come up with a temporary solution or to tell a false story to convince the senile'! (pp. 5–22, my italics!)

One person's experience

Jane Crisp is a university teacher of language and communication, literature, film and media, in Australia, and her mother has Alzheimer's disease. She found that by applying techniques and insights drawn from her own subjects, she was better able to understand her mother and facilitate conversation with her. She says that 'despite my mother exhibiting all the standard symptoms of the condition, I find that what she says continues to make good sense to me' (Crisp 1993). When she began to read the literature associated with dementia she found that it mostly concentrated on identifying what people get wrong, rather than on what they were still able to achieve. 'The research into the dysfunctions of language shows indirectly how long people with Alzheimer's disease are still able to use language to interact with others, even if they fail to perform the clinical tests set them correctly. This is not what is being studied though, *so tends to get ignored*' (my italics).

She then sets out some underlying strategies to encourage caregivers. The first one is that we should *value the fact that the person we care for is still interacting with us.* However advanced their dementia may be, always assume that they are still a real person and treat them as such 'even when their vocalisation is reduced to echoing words or to grunts and cries, they are still attempting to express themselves and to make contact with others'. The next stage is to forget about what is wrong with their response and to ask in what ways is it appropriate? That is, always be looking for something positive. Even when they make mistakes – in fact precisely because they make mistakes, we can see that certain basic rules of language are still operating. She points out that about 65 per cent of the 'wrong' answers to a question asking people to identify an object actually had some sort of association with that object, suggesting that the brain was functioning in a particular way not far short of how it should be functioning. So when a person uses an inappropriate word, ask yourself *what connection could the wrong word be expressing?* Linked to this is the strategy of asking if a sentence would make sense if we looked beyond the word that was being used to a more general category. So she suggests that we mentally add 'like this in some way' to what is being said.

Another tip is to ask if what the person is saying or doing makes sense if we relate it to something which might have happened to them in the past. We have to recognise that their sense of time may be different to our own, and they may no longer give us the clues that we need to be able to locate what they are saying in the 'correct' time zone. She stresses the importance of finding out their frame of reference and warns us against the unconscious imposition of our own. We can do this by simple questions, and by carefully listening.

A more difficult situation arises when the person tells us stories about themselves in which the present and the past are merged, as are actual things that have happened to them which are merged with things that other people have told them. 'It may help if we realise that these stories are very much like dreams, which seem to be a mixture of fact and fantasy, yet seem real enough when we are having them'. Many apparently untrue stories may become clearer to us if we ask ourselves if this is one character and place, or is it a combination of different characters and places which might be generally like this? Try to think of it more as a story, she says, and the person with dementia as the storyteller, and remember that telling a true story usually involves embroidering the facts a little in order to make it a good story and worth telling. She found that when her mother was engaged in this process, and when she was an active listener, it gave her mother some significance, and two powerful roles. She became a storyteller of a worthwhile story and also became the central character in the story too. 'Forget for the moment whether all the details are true or not. What value does the story have for its teller? Does it present them as important, worthwhile? Does it work through anxieties they might have? What more general message do the events give us? Do they stand in for something different but similar that is especially relevant to this person?'

Service and cost implications

In terms of service provision the implications of taking communication seriously are huge. If we were really convinced that it is possible to communicate, even to advanced stages and that, if it is possible, it is also desirable and necessary, then the implications for service provision would be far-reaching. We would invest more into one-to-one relationships with staff and there would be considerable training implications. As one Principal Officer put it in his reply to me:

> Communication is possible, but in the current economic climate it may not be possible in terms of staff hours to provide the time, patience, skill and commitment to communicate with people with dementia...I am concerned that there is no positive concern to elicit the views of the demented on the service being provided in case there are (and I suspect there are) many resource implications.

A similar awareness of the implications was conveyed by an Inspector who wrote:

> I think I might want to stress more strongly the consequences of not hearing what people with dementia are saying in so far as this is discriminatory in the extreme. The real issue here is time. My experience is that it can take weeks or months to begin to understand what one is being told. There are at least two consequences to this:

(a) the resource implications for service providers whose staff are usually very hard pressed and have insufficient time to devote to this, and

(b) the problem for demented people who have to wait the weeks or months it takes for their dissatisfactions to be understood

There are also important issues for ethnic minority sufferers who may revert to a language that is not English which needs to be addressed. Providers may need to seek expert help.

The deputy manager of a home for older people responded at length, and I will close this chapter with the little cameo that he presented:

I'm not sure that views of people with dementia can be elicited in a traditional question and answer way but I feel that people with dementia are so honest about their feelings and emotions that it is relatively easy to interpret their views by observing their behaviour and mood.

Recently I worked with a woman who was constantly looking for her babies (now in their 50s). She was in a permanent state of anxiety, wandering up and down corridors and trying to leave the building. All the staff struggled with this behaviour and nothing we did seemed to ease her anxiety. I then came across the ideas of Tom Kitwood which caused me to interpret the behaviour. We concluded that she was trying to express motherly feelings and we found that simple comments like 'I could really do with a cuddle' enabled the resident to express those feelings and reduce her anxiety. Later she found a doll on a display and began to talk to it, dress it, wash it, feed it. Some people struggled with the idea of an older woman 'playing' with a doll, but through it she was able to express all the feelings she needed to. No-one could observe her gentleness and tenderness and happiness with the doll without feeling moved. In her way, I feel she was telling us we were doing the right thing. Certainly her anxiety was dramatically reduced. An even stranger thing was evident – it appeared that her conversations with the doll were quite lucid and appropriate, whereas conversations with people were invariably difficult if not impossible to follow.

The implications for service provision are – sophisticated dementia care training for care staff and appropriate staffing levels.

Conclusions

It does seem that the opportunities for communicating depend to a large extent upon the belief of the person without dementia that communication is possible. Given that belief, then there invariably follows a determination to acknowledge the obstacles and problems to seek to find a way through them. Without such a conviction it is all too easy to conclude either that communciation is not possible, or that it is only a remote possibility. The implications for service provision are obvious – deny the possibility of communication and we increase our control over people and disempower them even further; it is a self-fulfilling stance.

CHAPTER 6

Disempowerment

> *People with dementia are not only disempowered by their illness, they are often disempowered by people's attitudes towards them. When people realise that what happens to them is independent of their responses they can 'learn helplessness'. This often happens in institutions. We need to be moving towards situations in which people are encouraged to have as much power over their lives as possible; this can be difficult for people with dementia, but there are so many ways in which they can be empowered if we are on the look-out for them.*

The person with dementia is often disempowered in two ways. First by the illness itself and, second, by other people's reactions to the illness and to the person concerned. The consultative document that I sent out to over a thousand people, asking for their comments put it this way:

> Not only are people having to cope with a debilitating illness, they are also confronted by a plethora of services and service providers. In this process they are often made 'objects' and their dignity and sense of worth is diminished. There is a process of disempowerment and disregarding, within which the failure to hear the voice of the person with dementia is one of the most persistent.

Robyn Yale (1993) is the project director of a study in California which seeks to provide support and information for people who have been diagnosed as suffering from Alzheimer's disease. She has set up many groups for people in which they talk to one another and express their concerns and fears. It is obvious from her work that early dementia patients, at least, have many issues to discuss when given the opportunity, and she says that 'it is essential that professionals be aware of biases which have dehumanised Alzheimer disease patients, for example regarding them as unable to express their thoughts and emotions'. This sense was reflected in a great many of the replies that I received to my document, and many people wrote in saying how the views of the person with dementia were consistently overruled, ignored or assumed not to exist. Typical was this comment from a senior nurse:

> At our home we work very hard to maintain personhood but we are often in a difficult situation as on many occasions social workers and family members seem to have more to say than the resident. In one recent instance, a gentleman was taken out of our care by his son and placed in a 'cheaper' homes despite the father stating that he was happy where he was. It is noticeable that we are advised to seek relatives' permission for residents to go out to different events and even then relatives can veto a decision that a resident has made. I know it is a difficult issue but I feel residents can give informed opinions on what they want and need provided time is spent with them and good communication skills used.

One officer in charge of a residential home went even further and said:

> Disempowerment seems to be mandatory! Often I have found that disempowerment begins within days of, or even prior to a diagnosis of dementia. Often by the time we are in contact with the client the person has ceased to try and regain the 'locus of control'.

Lubinski's (1991) view is that:

> Elderly individuals with dementia are among the most devalued members of our society, regardless of their lifelong characteristics and contributions…individuals who once fitted into the mainstream of society, demonstrating competence and productivity over their life span, now become marginal members within their immediate families and even more so within the larger social framework…the elderly demented individual bears the double stigma of age and mental handicap. (p.142)

It is important that we try to understand and appreciate the world of dementia; this is why it is crucial that we gain more understanding of what the experience is like. If we understand what the person is going through, if we can imagine what the world might be like from their standpoint, then it is more likely that our own attitudes might be more flexible, more tolerant and altogether more appropriate, but it is not easy.

The combination of a limited insight with engulfing feelings of anxiety, needing constant reassurance is an underlying feature of the person who feels the cognitive self slipping away…people in the earlier stages of brain failure are often embarrassed and caught out by their incapacity, fearful of being scolded, rejected or mocked…people with dementia seem to have difficulty in executing a plan…similarly incontinence, a particular trouble, is often less about bladder control than about the ability to interpret the signal and translate it into immediate action with foresight and hindsight about the effect of failing to do so. (Froggatt 1988, p.132)

Learned helplessness

Lubinski describes the condition of 'learned helplessness'. This is what occurs when a person perceives that events and outcomes are independent of their responses, and so they conclude that any further action is pointless. 'When demented persons perceive that their responses are futile, they stop responding' (p.142). When this happens, then the significant people around them do not expect the person to provide direct feedback, or to be able to perform capably, and the vicious circle of dependency is reinforced and the person is disempowered even more. Not expecting any feedback from the person with dementia, those around them assume a sort of monitoring role and begin to watch them closely to prevent potential harm, embarrassment or difficult situations. It is a spiralling process of low expectations and high dependency. What is happening is that clear signals are being sent out that no one expects the person with dementia to be able to participate meaningfully or competently, and so opportunities for interaction are reduced, and those responsible for the diminishing world for the person with dementia feel that their actions are justified by the results which emerge.

The more we expect from those who have dementia, the more opportunities we will provide for them to respond to. It is all a matter of treating the person with respect, as so many people wrote in explaining. If we fail to believe that the person with dementia is still a person in their own right, then we may easily fall into the habit of treating them as less than a person. The fact that the person may quietly accept this does not necessarily mean that they do not feel humiliated or disempowered, they may merely have retreated further into their own survival system. As Alison Froggatt (1988) pointed out, 'there is a distinction between the cognitive self which may be affected by memory loss and the experiencing feeling self which may be much less impaired, but hampered by an incapacity to verbalise' (p.133). One project manager in the field of mental health and learning disabilities wrote in with an example which sadly is not unique:

> When my father was in the local hospital ward for Alzheimer or dementia patients where clothes were laundered centrally, he wasn't always dressed in his own clothes. He was a big man and it was distressing for all of us on visiting him to see him wearing clothes which clearly didn't fit and served to take away the little dignity he had left.

One of the most frequent ways of disempowering people is to treat them as an object. This is as true in the research literature as it is in the caring field. In a much quoted passage, Cotrell and Schulz (1993) write:

> In the majority of research on Alzheimer's Disease, the afflicted person is viewed as a disease entity to be studied rather than someone who can contribute directly to our understanding of the illness and its course...the person with dementia is often relegated to the status of object rather than legitimate contributor to the research process...investigation has focused on cognitive functioning and patient management, with a notable absence of interest in patient awareness and in adaptation to increasing impairment and changing social status as a cause of psychiatric symptoms...one of the most common conditions in Alzheimer's disease is depression. (p.205)

This all ties in with the concept of personhood discussed in Chapter 3. There really does seem to be a fundamental difference between those who begin by assuming that the person with dementia has something to offer and those who begin by assuming that they are no longer capable of making a contribution. A clinical neuropsychologist who wrote in suggested that this divide might begin at an early stage, and that the person with dementia himself or herself might be part of the process which produces such a difference.

> Their first encounter with medical staff and diagnosis is often accompanied by words to the effect 'there is nothing we can do'. In the medical model this may be true at the moment. Socially, psychologically it is not true. Many of the effects of dementia are secondary to the actual disease process; the embarrassment amongst friends and the isolation this brings, the notion that one might as well give up and let others take over all decision making, the depression over the losses which dementia brings.

We are faced by a situation in which those who want to ignore the feelings and views of people with dementia can find sufficient reasons for doing so, and those who want to affirm their right to be consulted and to take their views into consideration can also provide reasons for doing so. It is not yet commonly accepted that the person with dementia has a viewpoint, nor is it commonly accepted that if they do communicate a viewpoint then this should be listened to and acted upon. In such a situation, the result is one of increased powerlessness for the person with dementia. A staff nurse wrote in commenting:

> In my experience the disempowerment of the individual is at the top of the list. As a professional I have seen numerous instances when clients do not want a particular course of action taken, but those handling the case nurses/doctors/social workers know that the client has no other option, therefore the client's wishes are ignored. For example, rehousing, placement into care, etc. This has always been a dilemma: what comes first, the client's safety or their wishes?

This is likely to be the case until we can bring about a change in the whole climate of dementia care as the sense of powerlessness goes back a long time, according to a director of nursing services who wrote.

> The main reason is, I believe, of historical nature. Previously, as soon as dementia was mentioned the person was normally institutionalised and thereafter became a 'victim' of these institutional regimes thereby increasing the deterioration of their condition. This can also happen when a person with dementia remains in their own home setting when spouse/families 'do' everything for them for the best of reasons in their opinion.

Institutionalisation

There has been a great deal written about the effects of institutions on people, and of hospitals in particular. Tom Kitwood (1990) speaks about the 'effects of institutionalisation *per se*, with its well-known tendency to deprive individuals of their former identity, and to reconstruct them within the institutional frame' (p.184). Oliver Sacks (1984), writing about his own experience of being a patient said

> I saw that one must be a patient, and a patient among patients, that one must enter both the solitude and the community of patienthood, to have any idea of what 'being a patient' means. (Quoted in Peloquin 1993a)

Sacks felt himself 'left out' of things; he saw people talking together and talking about him, but did not know what they were saying.'The hospital, in short, is a singular mixture, where freedom and bondage, warmth and coldness, human and mechanical, life and death, are locked together in perpetual combat' (1983). If the mentally alert and the highly respected can feel marginalised and powerless in a hospital setting, what must it be like for the more vulnerable? Suzanne Peloquin (1993a) describes a chilling scenario:

> An old woman with yellowed hair and failed hearing may not get an explanation because she is judged incomprehensing. A black man wearing tattered clothes may wait for hours because his time is judged less valuable. An unkempt teenager who reeks of liquor might face rough handling because her life is judged loathsome. Patients like these hear sharp demands to 'stay in line' because they are seen as having stepped beyond some value-laden boundaries set up by their practitioners. Although genuinely ill, these patients attract labels like *difficult* or *noncompliant* that rationalise the hidden bias of their helpers while mitigating their care. (p.834)

Many people wrote in describing their sense of grief when someone close to them was placed in a hospital setting, or in some form of residential care. There was a feeling that powerlessness was becoming all-pervasive. As one clinical psychologist commented, the key danger is that the outsider, the professional in the institution 'looks for and concentrates on what the person is *not* able to do. Assessment is of weaknesses rather than of strengths. Such lopsided concern has the effect of devaluing any remaining skills'. Karen Lyman (1989) notes that 'dependency is encouraged and acts of independence are either ignored or punished in long-term facilities' (p.602).

The dependence which is fostered by many nursing and residential homes limits the options for many people with dementia and this is particularly so in the case of physical exercise. This is commented on by Beck *et al.* (1992), who claim that a lack of exercise 'can deprive the cognitively impaired person of a sense of identity, leading to frustration, depression and resultant disruptive behaviour' (p.213).

Cotrell and Schulz (1993) speak of the twin experiences of *felt* stigma and *enacted* stigma. Felt stigma is when a person is embarrassed or ashamed because they have a particular illness. Enacted stigma is when people discriminate against or reject a person because of the consequences of their illness and many people with dementia may well have a fear of encountering such stigma. Alzheimer's disease, with its 'potential for producing intellectual incompetence, inevitably produces a changed status or identity, which can result in social unacceptability or inferiority' (p.206).

The plight of many people arriving in hospital or in different residential accommodation is well described by Ann Allison (1994), who writes:

> It helps if staff understand that much of the behaviour of these patients is a consequence of the fact that they basically feel lost and therefore stressed and frightened. They sometimes have no memory of how they got to the hospital, and no way of making sense of the experience. They are ill, bewildered and often upset. People they do not know call them names they do not expect and do things to them which they do not understand. (p.30)

It is the experience of many that when people with dementia are placed in residential accommodation alongside the cognitively intact, then there is often a considerable amount of discrimination. McGregor and Bell (1994) who run a specialist home for people with dementia have commented:

> In a mixed home, with frail elderly residents, people with dementia face continual failure, since they are regarded as a nuisance, unpleasant and anti-social. No-one wants them around. This destroys their self-confidence and their self image. It creates withdrawal, insecurity and depression...as professional carers it is our job to reverse this process and create a 'benign social psychology'. Our residents need to believe that they are valued and valuable, loved and appreciated, and that they do have something to offer the rest of us. (p.20)

Towards empowerment

If it is true that many people are left unheard and their wishes are not taken into consideration, and there is ample evidence to suggest that this is so, then it is also true to say that in many establishments great care is taken to try and empower people. There are many examples of good practice and quite a number of people wrote in with examples. The deputy manager of a home for older people wrote:

> One of our residents was empowered through attempts to really hear what she was saying. I don't know of any particular methods and would be pleased to hear about some. I think it probably stems from total listening and making huge attempts to interpret what people are saying/needing.
>
> I run a dementia care group (for care staff) and we produce dementia care plans through in-depth exploration, to find appropriate

approaches. We ask questions like 'what is the problem?', 'what is the person actually saying?', 'what else might this mean?' Recently, through adopting this approach a woman in her middle nineties changed from an antagonistic person who regularly hurled abuse at people to someone who was pleasant and thoughtful. She began insisting on turning the light out when she came out of the toilet, she became more interested in her appearance, she initiated conversation with others and became less territorial. Her demands were much less frequent, reasonable and appropriate. This did not happen all the time but it did seem to depend on who was on duty and who was using the correct approach. I believe our new approach enabled the resident to find her real self again, which was truly empowering.

Another example of empowerment comes from the manager of a residential home. It is just a small event, but can be held on to and cherished as one of those little things that can give meaning to life.

A resident who had very limited verbal communication went out shopping with her keyworker, to buy a new dress. The keyworker suggested this 'pretty red dress', the lady's reaction was one of total shock and she said 'Me? Red?' whilst shaking her head and throwing the dress aside, then turning to a blue one. The keyworker's reaction was as shocked as she was when she saw the resident's reaction to the red dress, for a person who had such limited communicative abilities. Involve people in all discussions on them, even facial expressions and body language gives them empowerment. We must learn to decipher.

Empowerment involves offering and respecting choices. These may be very small in themselves, but added together can enrich life. Having a choice about which clothes to put on, what to eat, or which chair to sit on is important. Having a choice about being involved in activities or not, or having a choice about whom to sit near, are all examples of ways in which people may be empowered.

For staff, promoting empowerment entails having good observational skills, and being able to interpret and assess. Thus in order to encourage empowerment there are implications for service provision. We need a skilled and trained workforce, we need more carers (formal or informal), for empowerment is time consuming, it being invariably quicker to make decisions for people than to allow them to make them for themselves, and, as one person wrote in, it involves role reversal: 'we have to adopt a minor role in all interactions, it is their views which are important'. This point was echoed by a project co-ordinator who reminds us that 'staff often need to be taught to "ask" rather than tell'. The importance of skilled observation was emphasised in the Cotrell and Schulz (1993) article referred to earlier. They write:

> In the advanced stages of dementia, language deficits limit the individual's ability to communicate through propositional language and the person's psychosocial needs can only be inferred from behaviour. This makes effective patient care more difficult. Accurate interpretation of behaviour is important for effectively dealing with the individual's isolation created by the loss of communication. How do we know what the individual wants or needs?...Much needs to be learned about the feelings and desires of human beings who are unable to express themselves'. (p.208)

Perhaps, in the light of the previous chapter, we would want to soften those final words 'unable to express themselves', but the thrust of their statement remains; accurate observation is needed if we are really intent on empowering people.

A conflict of interest?

A charge nurse sent in the following comment:

> There is an expectation among society at large that people with dementia should be 'looked after', that is, shielded from society, from all risk. The emphasis on quantity as opposed to quality of life is usually at odds with the views of people with dementia themselves.
>
> One mildly demented man once told me whilst acknowledging that he was at risk because of his failing faculties, that he would rather live for three weeks at home than for three years in care. His relatives opposed this view.
>
> The relatives' view is a philosophy supported by most professionals, either because they share this perception of the person with dementia's needs or because they fear the consequences should a dementia victim in their care suffer misadventure because he or she was not protected from risk. The implications of this are immense. If the wishes of the dementia sufferers are complied with, enormous numbers of them will remain in their own homes in preference to accepting institutional care. This will require a radical shift in society's expectations or an increase in funding of support care that would probably be beyond the means of a government with a genuine commitment to the care of the sick. Or both.

This tension, or conflict of interests was made very clear by a research fellow and counsellor who wrote in.

> Empowerment is now a central theme for social workers and dementia throws down one of the greatest challenges. The question of empowerment and rights versus risks comes up again and again in my work with social work students. One of the greatest dilemmas for social workers faced with a person with dementia and their family is 'Who is my client?' I am frequently asked by social workers and students what they should do when there is a conflict of interest between the person with dementia and his or her carers. Historically, I think, we have tended to collude with the family, thinking that they know what is best for their relative. One of the new challenges is to respond to the needs of the person with dementia, as verbalised by the person themself. New research shows us that the person with dementia can still hold an opinion about what they want and what they feel is best for them.

A senior physiotherapist spelled out the dilemma of people working in the field:

> We constantly strive to empower our clients. Obtaining their views is at best time consuming and it is sometimes not possible, so we end up taking on primarily the view of the main carer (which is not always the client's). I think also there can be some conflict between our desire to 'keep the clients safe' whilst respecting their wishes – for example – if someone is at risk at home of burning themselves and cannot be 'made safe', how should we respond? They may refuse Meals on Wheels and want to cook for themselves – should we allow this if they are at risk? Implication – effective team working will help us to work respectfully with clients and carers since we are accountable to each other. Also, the 'difficult situations' are better managed when discussed within a team.

A sister/manager of a day centre for people with dementia admitted that service planners do not always have the necessary time or skills to listen to people with dementia and so, when services are planned, they are often planned to meet the needs of carers. One daughter wrote in 'my father has *not* been empowered, for his needs and those of his carer (my mother) are at opposite ends of the spectrum'.

Thus it is important for purchasers and particularly for service providers to recognise the power relationships which exist between people with dementia and their carers. If this is not acknowledged then it can mean that the person with dementia may not be allowed to participate in discussions about care. It can mean that the responses which are given when consultations take place and the needs which surface are those of the carer rather than of the person with dementia. It can be much easier for service providers to consult with relatives and, as an assistant director of community liaison warned, 'it is important that carers do not collude with service providers and purchasers and that they ensure that the person with dementia's needs are heard and taken on board'. This is not to minimise the genuine needs of carers. There are real problems for many carers, and they need help and support, but we need to be able to differentiate between their needs and the needs of the person with dementia, and to recognise whose needs are being met at any one time and by any particular provision. Often, of course, the needs of both may be met at the same time – but this should not be taken for granted.

Advocacy

In recent years the idea of advocacy has been gaining ground in a number of areas. This is where a skilled 'outsider' takes the time and trouble to find out what the person is really wanting, and explains or communicates what the possible options might be. They can act as an intermediary between the person with dementia and the professionals, and seek to ease the process of communication between them. A social work team leader commented that the most common form of disempowerment arose from a failure to treat the person with respect, the 'objectification of the person to non-person status', and recommended that the development of user-sensitive advocacy schemes should be promoted. This idea is still in its infancy, but is obviously a possible way forward. A member of an advisory team for older people commented:

> The issue of advocacy on behalf of people with dementia is clearly important. There is a need for policy and guidelines on this to make sure that those used in the role of advocate really do have the interests of the older person at heart. If we do not have access to a formal advocate (because this role is not very well developed in services for older people) then are we formally testing out the adequacy of individuals to take on the role?

Perhaps there is scope here for some developmental work. I am aware that only in a few places does advocacy take place with people with dementia, but have not been able to find sufficient material describing and assessing how it is done.

Conclusion: Empowerment is not just an idea

It is important to stress that people can be empowered in a whole manner of small ways and that these, when added together, can be powerful indicators of change. To talk about empowerment is not to 'philosophise about an idea', but to turn words into practical actions which honour and respect people. One person wrote in expressing considerable concern about the danger of 'empowerment' becoming an 'in word' and thus a failure to make changes in practice.

> My gut feeling on this issue is the possible danger of getting bogged down in the processes and structures rather than looking at indicators of empowerment and outcomes. For instance, the need to look at what the client had been empowered to do or experience or change in their life. I think that Kitwood's dimensions of *well being* deserve a lot of attention and testing...

One risk and consequence for services is, I fear, rejection. I have come across some notable instances. I heard that there was an attempt to introduce a home help to a client who clearly needed some very practical support and/or emotional support, and who rejected it when it was put to them (in an 'abstract' way). They were asked if they needed a home help. The same person clearly enjoyed their chat with me. It appeared that if anyone had first introduced the home help as a person to engage in conversation, and then ask if they would be interested in their coming again, it is clear that there would have been a different response. This is a concrete example of focusing too much on the abstract nature of empowerment (informed consent, in this case) as opposed to the more concrete empowerment when related to a specific relationship situation and the consequence.

CHAPTER 7

A Sense of Time and Pace

We need to slow down when we are with people with dementia; we need to adapt to their pace and time-scale rather than expect them to adopt ours. It takes time to get into a 'communicative mode' and to rush invariably makes the meeting counter-productive. We need to acknowledge the pressures of time that we experience and learn how to deal with them. We have to 'make time for communication' and learn how to become 'active listeners', which can be quite demanding and difficult.

The role of volunteers as an additional resource is discussed.

Often, difficulties encountered when communicating can be attributed to the pace of the interaction. Communicating with a person with dementia can be a slow process. We must be prepared to devote an adequate and appropriate amount of time to this task. Very often metaphors may be used, which need to be interpreted. Not having enough time, and therefore making little progress is not the same as saying that the person is unable to communicate. Communication may be extremely difficult because, for whatever reason, we are not able to devote an adequate amount of time to that specific task.

This was another key area that I set out in my consultative document and I asked people to say whether, in their experience, pressures of time had made it more difficult for them to communicate with people with dementia. I also wondered if people had any suggestions to make as to how service providers might be able to reach a balance between respecting the time and pace of the person with dementia, whilst at the same time providing an economical service.

It seems that this is a crucial area, and I wondered how appropriate to our setting were the observations of Suzanne Peloquin (1993b), writing from her North American context:

practitioners face a major quandary when their patients' needs for time and compassion compete with the institution's need to prosper. When high regard falls to those who treat most patients or accumulate the most billable units of time, moments spent noticing, listening or communicating are harder to justify. (p.940)

Few people would use the same language in our context, but there is a widespread feeling of frustration that perceived staffing shortages and pressures on time mean that care is not given in the way that most people would like to give it, and communication is one of the first casualties of working under such pressure. Of all the replies that I received, over 200 in number, only one person replied that in their situation they did not feel this sort of pressure. A day care worker commented that

> due to excellent staffing levels we find pressure of time not a problem – communication with carers, support group meetings, care plans (with updated aims and issues) and regular reviews, with client's views recorded, all take place.

This contrasts vividly with the pleas for more time which came from so many respondents, as illustrated by this comment from a development nurse in dementia services:

> rushing any conversation with a person with dementia, or rushing off when you know they haven't understood without coming back to clarify the statement is tantamount to abuse. Perhaps this may be a controversial comment, but on the basis of that belief I would go on to say that people with dementia are being abused on hospital wards up and down the country. In making that sweeping accusation I have to also admit that I can offer no suggestions that would make an immediate difference to this.

That is the crux of the issue. If we know that care is not being provided to the level that we would wish, and if we know that in the area of communication there is so much that needs to be done to improve things, then what is to be the way forward? First, we need to go back to the basic issue of whether we believe that communication is, in fact, possible. We need to reflect on the issues raised in Chapter 4. We need to acknowledge just how much work the people with dementia very often put into their effort to communicate with us. As one person commented to me, 'if everyone put as much effort into trying to understand the communication as the person with dementia puts into communicating, it might be better achieved'. We need to discover new ways of allowing ourselves to make the very most of the amount of time that is available to us. There are two issues here; one concerns the absolute amount of time at our disposal and how effectively we use it, the other concerns the amount of time that *ought* to be available, and there may be ways of working towards enlarging it.

Kitwood (1990) gives us some helpful clues as to how we might approach the process:

> We need to slow down our thought processes, to become inwardly quiet, and to have a kind of poetic awareness; that is, to look for the significance of metaphor and allusion rather than pursuing meaning with a kind of relentless tunnel vision. (p.51)

We have to allow the person to get into the right mode, and not assume that we can suddenly move up to him or her and begin a conversation. As one carer put it, 'I have learned through interaction with my father that I need to allow him a lot of time to get into a communicative situation'. This needs to be borne in mind when communication has to take place about being in a certain place by a certain time. Getting to a doctor's surgery, or being ready to be picked up by a minibus can be major problems for a carer, and we do not yet know what these times of pressure mean to the person with dementia. What is clear though is that we should not impose our own frame of reference onto them; the whole process has to be much more sensitive, relaxed and subtle.

This is not always easy for staff when they have many other jobs to do and must work to a tight schedule. There is an enormous temptation to expect the person with dementia to adapt to the pressures and routines of the service, rather than the other way round. What often happens therefore is that the 'jobs' get done and taking time to develop communication is seen as a luxury, or something to be done when there are a few minutes spare. As Gemma Jones (1992) reflects

> these results are not surprising if one realises that it takes a great deal of energy and time to speak to persons who are difficult to communicate with, and, when staffing levels have been pared down to a minimum, staff feel pressures to become task-oriented rather than communication-oriented. These orientations unfortunately are still seen as distinct rather than complementary. (p.86)

Increasingly staff are being encouraged to see that the tasks can in fact be vehicles for conversation, and that they may be used to provide a non-threatening context within which communication might be encouraged. As one senior nurse for mental health commented:

> The best way to ensure that the communication talked about here is carried out is to *write it in a care plan* [my italics]. Once this is done, you start educating staff into the idea that psychological care is equally as important as physical care and not something you tack onto the end. If you create this idea and adopt a non-institutional approach you find the beds are made and towels etc. are put out quickly in between conversations and not made the *major task* [her emphasis] of the morning.

Pressures of time

The fact remains that many staff feel themselves to be under a great deal of pressure and this mitigates the possibilities of being able to provide the 'dream service' which was mentioned in the previous chapter. It is perhaps worth quoting a number of the comments about pressures of time and pressures of staffing. These suggest that there are both overall problems and also problems of management, for whatever the staffing levels are, the challenge remains to provide as effective and as individualised a service as possible. The quotations here are almost taken at random from the replies that came in.

- Yes, pressures of time do impact on the amount of time needed to communicate with a person… I think it is vital that supervisors/workload managers provide 'permission' for practitioners to take some extra time to 'unpack' what a client is saying to us.
- Low staffing levels makes it very difficult to devote as much time as would be preferable – this in turn generates frustration and agitation.
- Most people in the health services are very short of time and this does lead to communication problems.
- Staff also need to be respected/trained and empowered, and this is harder where numbers are low.
- The services we give do not help staff to develop a close relationship which enhances understanding. Social workers have no time for slowly working with someone; residential staff necessarily work shifts; *everything is stacked against the person with dementia* [my italics].
- [Staff] do not have the time and frequent misinterpretations occur.

- 'People haven't got time to talk to me now because it takes such a long time. I've never been an over-volulopus [sic] person. I'm feeling I'm getting more silent.'

- Time is the main difficulty in communication. In General Practice the only way to deal with this is by delegating to a professional such as the Health Visitor or Practice Nurse who may be able to commit more time to the communication process.

- Many physical and behavioural activities must take precedence over communication if one is to be honest and practical.

- With the pressure on resources it is difficult to know how to allocate more time, but it is important that we try to do so.

- Our staffing levels mean pressures of time are a recurrent problem which can leave staff feeling frustrated and residents psychologically damaged.

- People with dementia on general hospital wards rarely get the care they need because no one has the time or skill to sit and discuss needs.

- Pressures on staff time have clearly affected their ability to respond appropriately to the user's own time and pace.

- Pressure of time or lack of effective time can be destructive.

These comments come from just about every part of the service delivery side, from planners to managers, from consultants to care assistants, and many more examples could be given. The overriding theme seems to be that there just is not enough time to do the job properly. There is also an awareness that sometimes doing the job inadequately can be counter-productive. Although it is perhaps worth noting that sometimes the arguments about pressure of time and shortage of staff can be used to conceal other issues, as one particular ward sister pointed out:

> It is greatly over-used as an excuse by some nurses who appear to feel safer if not involved with the feelings and needs of the client with dementia. Staff training which allows the carer to see for themselves that task-orientated work produces ill-being in our clients and a boring and thankless job for the carer. It is then seen as the carer's responsibility to change nursing practice to one which is of benefit to the client's needs. I feel that we need to show, as managers, that we have the time to care for the carers.

Ways forward

The situation does not have to be one of demoralisation and failure. There are many instances of good practice, and there are several ways in which the problems can be tackled. Training is one of them. Many staff need to have greater confidence in their ability to communicate with people with dementia. Knowing that they are embarking upon a difficult process which requires skills which can be learned, can make it a rewarding challenge for them and bring a greater sense of job satisfaction. Management needs to ensure that time is allowed for communication, and encouragement given to staff for them to have confidence to know that time spent relating to people is mainstream care, and is not a diversion from other, more important tasks.

We need to discover the art of listening creatively. If we are to move at the time and pace of the person with dementia, we have to allow them to set that pace and not impose it upon them.

> Active listening is, by definition, a nonpassive role. The listener is required to be attentive to all that is said and unsaid, and to be prepared to offer unconditional positive regard throughout all interactions. This type of listening is a difficult role to maintain for any length of time…it was not always easy to listen at this level. It was found to be tiring and draining, the emotions displayed by the informants themselves were often negative, powerful and intense. Occasionally these feelings transferred themselves to the researcher, who during these times felt helpless, vulnerable and forlorn. (Mills and Coleman 1994, p.214)

Staff who engage with people will also very often find it demanding and difficult. It is all the more important to persevere when the temptation is to move away and talk to someone else. We can but imagine what it might mean to the person with dementia if people consistently move away from them when they fail in their efforts to communicate. The experience of the person who would be a listener is well described by C K Li (1993).

> To acknowledge that we don't really know, to be able to tolerate 'not knowing', requires enormous courage and humility…perhaps we are too keen to help; we are in a hurry to produce changes, to achieve insights. Listening is too time consuming…only with an attitude of silence could we hear clearly what the patient *and I* are saying. (p.9)

People often seem to need permission to sit alongside, and to move at the speed and timing of the person with dementia, they need to know that it is very often the mere fact that this is happening that is important – more important than what actually emerges in these times of togetherness. What emerges may or may not make sense, but the fact that someone has given the time, unconditionally, is the characteristic of good care, and is a sign that the person is taken seriously and is deemed to be important.

Volunteers as an additional resource

Quite a number of services are finding that limited resources are encouraging them to look elsewhere and many people wrote in describing their use of volunteers. These ranged from seeing volunteer help as a temporary stopgap measure in the face of a staffing shortage to developing long-term partnership arrangements with the voluntary sector. A nurse wrote:

> Caring volunteers are the best answer for serving those with dementia who need more time for communication to satisfactorily take place.

Whilst a carer made this observation:

> All too often I have seen pressure of time rob sufferers of essential stimulation that comes from talking with caring staff about their interests etc. Invariably the pressure of time is caused by staff shortages, but sometimes too by lack of appreciation of the importance of stimulation and personal contact with familiar people. Adequate regular staff, reinforced with 'befrienders' or relatives or friends seems to be a solution.

The Head of Joint Planning in one area wrote that:

> it is very difficult to continue with everyday life and find time for communication. Ideally it should be an area where the statutory and voluntary sectors work well together, i.e. nursing staff may get distracted by the phone etc., whereas a volunteer worker can hopefully concentrate on one person for a reasonable length of time.

Another way forward and one advocated by quite a number of people was to use untrained staff and to give them some responsibilities for sitting and talking to people – 'carefully selected unqualified staff would probably be quite quickly trained to play this sort of role' suggested a clinical psychologist, and several others made a similar point. I was interested to note a comment by a manager – 'use of trained volunteers or *allowing* relatives to do more can help alleviate the difficulty of not enough time' [my italics]. It does seem that relatives are so often left in a rather ambiguous situation by many service providers. In literally thousands of comments that I received during the course of my project, I could count on one hand those which suggested that relatives might be some sort of co-workers in dementia care. Now I realise that perhaps for many people this was merely stating the obvious, but I suspect that not enough creative thinking is being done to see how we might harness the love and commitment of relatives into a rather more creative force.

I am concerned that whilst much of the literature points out that listening is a skilled and demanding task, so many people seem to think that the answer might be in using the untrained staff in an establishment or in bringing in willing volunteers. There seem to be two sorts of process envisaged, both necessary and complementary, and one should not be seen as diminishing the need for the other. There is a great need for people to spend time alongside the person with dementia; perhaps a basic training might help them to feel confident enough to do this, but there is also a need for skilled engagement by people who are trained to pick up the various nuances and who fit into an overall care scheme, and can feed back the progress or the difficulties that any person is experiencing at any particular time.

It is a mistake to think that volunteers are, by definition, unskilled. Many of the volunteers that some establishments use bring a wide range of skills and are extremely sensitive. Many voluntary services, day care centres or sitting services, for example, rely upon volunteers and many of them are well trained and do excellent skilled and supportive work. Indeed, without their input, a great many of our services would fold up. What is needed is to ensure that there is a comprehensive training and support package, and for every service which uses volunteers to have a clearly defined strategy for their use and careful management to ensure that creative work is undertaken and that the various institutions or services are not merely 'warehousing' the people with dementia.

Untrained and unmanaged volunteers are of little use, but volunteers can be trained and then, if allocated *on a generous time scale*, can make an invaluable contribution to the 'being alongside' which is so important in dementia care. They have the great advantage of not needing to be goal orientated in this particular setting, and they can 'idle in neutral' as one person put it. Certain services, particularly residential and day care services, could be thinking in terms of recruiting an adequate supply of volunteers so that perhaps every person with dementia could have someone's attention for two or three hours a day. As one professional woman told me:

I'm useless when I'm in work mode in terms of relating to mum. I have to have switched off first and have to adopt her time-scale. Two or three hours are the minimum worthwhile togetherness stint.

Engaging volunteer help could make a significant difference to patterns of care, but it needs to be undertaken skilfully and sensitively and should be seen as a positive development rather than as a stopgap measure. There are useful guidelines on volunteering available from Volunteer Development Scotland, the UK Volunteer Forum, or local volunteer agencies. Attention would need to be given, of course, as to how feedback between volunteers and staff was handled, because there could be dangers of staff missing out on valuable contact time and also being unaware of how relationships and communications were developing.

Is it possible?

A principal officer for the elderly/physically disabled made this comment:

Adequate time has to be devoted to the person with dementia and what is more important, if possible, is that there should be a consistency in the person involved with the sufferer. I am afraid if this is to be achieved it looks as if it would be quite impossible to provide an economical service.

A project manager whose father was in long-stay care wrote:

when conversation and understanding became more difficult, I found in the early days that he would eventually home into me and I could get some response. It required a lot of patience and time. I often felt that even if he didn't understand what was being asked him, e.g. 'sit down Dad', the way it was said and the approach often got the desired result. Once I observed my father being tugged by a nurse to sit down – his reaction was to pull away because, I suspect, he was frightened and didn't know what was happening. I took over and with a gently, gently approach got him to sit down… I think it is difficult to find a balance between respecting the time and pace of people with dementia whilst at the same time providing an economical service.

A timely word of warning came from a Social Services Inspector:

The point about service provision is *effectiveness* and cost-effectiveness, not economy. Dementia is an expensive illness to care for if done properly. If rushed, it is counter-productive and the service is ineffective in meeting needs.

Conclusion

There is clearly quite a tension between trying to provide a service which operates according to the sense of time and pace of the person with dementia, and which meets the budgetary requirements set down for it. This is not the same thing as saying that spending more money would automatically improve services, or that services cannot be good and effective even though financially hard-pressed. It does appear, however, that a great many people working in this field feel that they are unable to provide the sort of care which they would ideally like to provide, because of the pressures of time and other limited resources. One of the first casualties, when working under such pressure, is having the time and space just to 'be' with a person; yet we know, that if we really want to communicate with people with dementia, this will take a considerable amount of time and cannot be rushed. At present, in order to provide services for people with dementia, it seems that it is necessary to limit the opportunities to develop effective communication, and thereby limit the quality of those services. This does not mean that the person with dementia does not have a voice, but it may mean that, as a society, we are not yet prepared to pay for listening to it.

CHAPTER 8

The Value of 'Life Story'

If we cannot identify ourselves, it is helpful to know what we have come from. Similarly with dementia; it is a good help in the process of communication if we can understand something about the background and life of the person before dementia has occurred. Autobiography, oral history, reminiscence, life story and life review are all possible ways of discovering the background and 'story' of the person, and enabling them to 'own' their particular history. 'You can climb up a family tree and see the vista from there,' said one person with dementia.

People build up patterns of behaviour during their life, and they often retain their behaviour patterns during their time of illness. It helps our approaches, and our attempts to communicate, if we can appreciate these patterns.

His tundra'd mind sprouts leaflets
    here and
    causes me to stare
    in new awareness of the man
    he must have been.
    Where he now
        struggles
            to retain
such meager lichen to his brain
    he must have raised
    rare orchids
    years ago   (Senile 1979–80)

It does not matter that, as a young girl growing up in Boston, Massachusetts, she helped to raise her seven brothers and sisters and that she took care of her elderly mother. It does not matter that she was once able to fix plumbing, hang wallpaper and prepare a full dinner every night, while keeping six kids out of major trouble. It does not matter that she could once swim faster than anyone in her family, that she secretly yearned to be a basketball star, that her late husband considered her the most beautiful woman he'd ever seen... (Kantrowitz 1989, p.46)

Another area that I wrote about in my consultative document was that concerning the importance of people's life story. I suggested that

communication is often assisted by rooting it within the life-context and history of the person with dementia, and in this way it is often possible to discover their views and preferences. Ability to communicate may be related to their ability to communicate before they had dementia. We need to know about their earlier personality and approach to life. Good dementia care is related to the whole person and not just to the 'area of need'.

I invited people to share any insights they might have as to how service provision might be affected if we could set our communication within the life-context of the person with dementia.

Mills and Chapman (1992) observed that:

Many of us who work with confused elderly people would agree that our knowledge of their past lives, as opposed to the diagnosis and progress of their illness, is inclined to be somewhat sparse...if these patients are seen as the sum total of their problems then the outlook is bleak. We need to see the person behind the dementia. (p.27)

A consultant psychiatrist wrote in saying that he was 'appalled by the lack of *personal* knowledge about some old people with dementia in residential and nursing homes', a point that Faith Gibson (1991) has also stressed:

Staff have acknowledged their abysmal ignorance of the person as a person in terms of knowledge about their past history. To say that little more was known about some of these people in care than was known about Jewish refugee children fleeing from the Nazi Holocaust who arrived in Britain with only a label around their necks, is only a slight exaggeration. Despite all the rhetoric about admission policies, admission practices are still all too often grossly inadequate especially when it comes to detailed knowledge about the person's past. (p.10)

If that is one end of the spectrum, there is a growing awareness of a different approach and, increasingly, service providers are being encouraged to see people within their life-context, and they are recognising that communication becomes a distinct possibility when we are more alive to the person with dementia as a living person with a history and with all sorts of interesting experiences and achievements. A hospital sister wrote of the effectiveness of this approach:

> by using a life history we have been able to provide activities relevant to the clients' needs, maintained respect and the individuality of the person. Care plans have then included discharge plans. We have effectively discharged from hospital three long-stay patients who had 'been given up on long since'. These people are now independent of hospital care and seem happy.

That is an unusual case, but a great many people commented on the value, indeed upon the necessity of getting to know the story of the person and of then delivering services which were appropriate to the person that they had discovered. It is still probably an ideal to suppose that everyone who comes into some form of care is treated in this way, but nevertheless the importance of life history work is gaining much greater acceptance now. A development nurse in dementia services wrote that

> one of my objectives for our unit is that every patient will have a life story within two weeks of admission, by the end of next year. This will then be used to help improve communication between next of kin and staff, and patient and staff. It will hopefully then be carried over to the next place of care (residential home etc.). This will enable continuity of care for the person with dementia and hopefully a strengthening of links between the hospital and the community can also be achieved.

Another comment from a residential home echoed the value of this approach.

> Knowledge of the narrative of the other *is* knowledge of the other. I think it is impossible to communicate with clients if the life story is unknown. Knowing their stories makes it possible for me to provide prompts and cues so that we can have an effective and meaningful conversation. This enables the enhancement of well-being and personhood. Returning their story to them seems to aid short periods of rementia. Good dementia care is then based on clearly expressed need through the story and through periods of lucidity.

The work is not without its lighter side, as a senior occupational therapist revealed:

care managers do endeavour to discover what they can about earlier life events as these do help understanding communication. A colleague of mine once interviewed an elderly lady who had once run a brothel and realised that she was being interviewed as a possible worker!

In a study done in America (Pietrukowicz and Johnson 1991), the attitudes of nursing staff to a resident were studied when some of them had been given a page of life history in the patient's notes and others had received notes without any life history. The research found that the staff who had read the life history thought that the resident was more capable of interacting with others, contributing socially and setting goals and adapting, than did the staff who had not read any life history. It would thus appear that, apart from anything else, the inclusion of life history notes affects the attitude of mind which the staff person brings to bear upon the person when they meet them.

Different approaches

There are a number of different terms used to describe slightly different approaches to life story, and it is perhaps helpful to recognise these distinctions. *Autobiography* is where the subject is the sole author and is an attempt to provide a comprehensive account of a life. *Oral history* is mainly done in groups, whose main concern is the retrieval of past experiences and its recording or preservation. *Reminiscence* is when groups share memories with the intention of understanding each other, or a shared situation, or with the aim of producing some change in their current lives. *Life story* is an individual approach to setting out a person's life, and it usually has some form of physical outcome, usually (although not necessarily) in the form of a scrapbook or something similar. *Life review* is the process of going over a person's life with a view to understanding or 'unpacking' certain events or significant people or situations; it does not have a physical outcome.

The two most common approaches used in working with people with dementia are reminiscence and life story.

LIFE STORY

Charles Murphy (1994) in a very useful publication on life story work says that it

> involves looking back on the past, usually on a one-to-one basis. It does not set out to resolve past problems or present ones (life review), although this may be an outcome. Similarly it does not aim to offer the information recovered for public or communal consumption (oral history), although again this may be the outcome. (p.4)

He then goes on to give reasons why people develop and use life story work in the context of dementia care, including:

- to gain a greater understanding of the person that they care for
- to find explanations in the past for things that are happening today
- to have something to pass on to the family carer when the individual moves on from the home care project, day centre or residential home
- to have something to pass on to the next 'service', which offers them an extra dimension to the person coming into care
- to help deliver better, more personalised care to the individual
- to orientate the individual to his/her present life
- to offer the person with dementia a failure-free fun activity
- to offer the individual a chance to give something back
- to give the family carer a sense of involvement and achievement through collecting life story material, and to give them something to do which they can share with their relative
- to observe and monitor changing needs
- to help the family carer to remember the many and varied aspects of the life and character of the person with dementia, and
- to have something for workers to remember the person by when they are no longer in their care.

One past carer wrote:

> With my mother we produced a 'This is your life' photo album. It was a prized possession, shared with every visitor. She herself used it as a memory jogger – it allowed strangers an insight into her background and allowed communication with less expenditure of effort on her part and retained her memories for longer than would have been otherwise.

Knowledge of a person's past can very often help us to understand their present situation with greater clarity. For instance a senior nurse for mental health commented that

> we find much repetitive behaviour can be traced and understood by reading life histories. For example, one lady who knelt on the floor smoothing the carpet for hours on end turned out to be a dressmaker and, if given a sheet, would line it up perfectly, with great satisfaction.

Similarly, a speech therapist with older people commented that

> it encourages professionals to view people with dementia as adults
> with a life history of experience and skills that may still be relevant
> and used in their daily lives to empower them. It helps to view the
> whole person and to hypothesise about actions we may not have
> understood before.

John Killick recounts a lovely phrase which occurred in one of his conversations with a person with dementia, 'You can climb up a family tree and see the vista from there'.

In some areas there are good community care support structures set up, and often in these situations the people who visit may well have shared the same local environment and culture, and perhaps even have a common history with the person with dementia. This could be true in more rural areas in particular and, as a respondent from one of the Scottish isles wrote, 'in our situation many staff have known the clients all their lives and can "tap-in" appropriately'. Another comment from rural Scotland made this point:

> In our area it helps a lot if the carer can speak Gaelic (my mother
> reverted back to Gaelic in her latter years). It will always help if the
> carer has the same background and knows the area and the way of
> life. This is especially true when it comes to religion. TV or other
> activities on a Sunday which the patient isn't used to because of
> Sabbath observances can be very upsetting and there is a need to make
> sure that those with a religious faith have an opportunity to express
> this either by being able to take part in services or listening to tapes
> etc.

I am reminded of one home that I visited regularly where one of the residents was a Roman Catholic who was in the habit of going to church each morning. For the whole of the time that she was in the home there had been no visit from a priest and she had taken part in no religious observance. Discussing it with the staff I discovered that they just had not known.

Murphy (1994) warns against assuming that there must always be a physical end product in life story work. It is not a task to be achieved, but a process to be valued. Nor should we be overly concerned with *facts* and *truth*. What is important is what the person wishes to share, and if we cannot fully understand the images they use or the information which is given, it is better to take it on trust, or on hold, until we can we better understand. The fact that the person presents material in the way that they do is itself a significant factor which we may understand better as time goes on.

Some establishments complete a *social history form*, which is a similar though perhaps smaller exercise than compiling a life story book. Mills and Chapman (1992) comment that when this is completed by the patient and primary carer, it

> can be viewed as a pleasurable and enjoyable activity. It would be appropriate as an activity and task at home, in a day centre, residential unit or hospital. A completed copy of the social history could then become part of the patient's files and would then be useful in enabling existing and future carers to communicate with, and have some understanding of, the elderly person with dementia. (p.30)

REMINISCENCE

Reminiscence is the process whereby past events get relived, and people often become quite involved. It is more than storytelling, it is a recalling of feelings and attitudes. It used to be regarded somewhat negatively and people were urged not to get 'bogged down' in the past, but in recent years it has been perceived as having considerable therapeutic merit. Faith Gibson (1991) is one of the great facilitators and exponents of this type of work. Speaking of her involvement in it she said:

> It has been a genuine journey of discovery, venturing into a landscape which in some ways seems familiar, but in others, constantly changing…it is important to say that my understanding of [it] shifts each time I reminisce with individuals or groups, with people who may have good memories, or poor memories. Each time I listen to old people tell me how it used to be for them, and each time I listen to people telling me about their own experience of reminiscence work, my understanding grows and my excitement about what we are doing is revitalised. (p.1)

It has been said that reminiscence work helps people to use the then and there of life to enrich the here and now, and Murphy (1994) lists a number of reasons for doing it, including:

- ◦ to give feelings of belonging
- ◦ to relay history and wisdom to a younger generation
- ◦ to develop relationships
- ◦ to leave a legacy to friends and extended family members
- ◦ to preserve identity
- ◦ to maintain self-esteem

- for therapeutic reasons, such as the resolution, reorganisation and reintegration of life events
- as a preparation for death
- as a form of self-expression, and
- as a way of communicating feelings.

Gibson (1994) has written that

> it is wide-ranging and critical. It emphasises the importance of communication, of being able to tell one's own unique life story and have it heeded and respected by others. This obviously presents a special challenge to those who seek to listen to people with dementia. (p.25)

A clinical neuropsychologist wrote in saying:

> The most exciting outcome [of knowing a person's life story] may be the use of previous experiences and reminiscence about them to establish views on current decisions. It would require the drawing of parallel between the past and the present, but would at least take advantage of relatively preserved memory for past events. For example, if a person with dementia had cared for their parents, then asking them to talk about how they cared for their mother, the things they did for her, what they felt was important, might allow us to draw parallels concerning what they would like for themselves. Based on 'do as you would be done by', but in reverse. Finding out about family traditions and rituals from the past could allow the recreation of those traditions in the present.

The sister/manager of a day care centre also felt that knowing more about a person's past was important is providing a more appropriate form of care in the present:

> Yes, knowledge of a sufferer's past history can give an indication of topics for conversation, their likes and dislikes, ideas for preferred recreational activities etc. People who have disliked socialising in the past will probably find the experience of a day care centre very frightening. However, they may accept a 'sitter' in their own home.

A theoretical diversion

When people have an illness which produces dementia, the person who becomes ill is the person who has developed over the years. All the experiences, good and bad, that made the person who they are are brought into the new situation and may, or may not, be remembered. Some people grow into difficult old people and others grow old pleasantly and gracefully; this is true whether or not they are ill. Having dementia can seem to exaggerate some of the characteristics of people and it certainly can remove some of the social restraints that we all exercise on different parts of our behaviour. The people who come into our care are people who have been fashioned and moulded by their experiences of life, and retelling some of those experiences can sometimes be distressing for them. By skilful listening, and with appropriate training, it may be possible to help people resolve some of the issues in their life which have been repressed and denied over the years.

Bowlby (1988) reminds us how patterns of behaviour are built up and these are the patterns which can sometimes become more apparent when a person grows and has dementia.

> ...a secure child is a happier and more rewarding child to care for and is less demanding than an anxious one. An anxious ambivalent child is apt to be whiny and clinging; whilst an anxious avoidant child keeps his distance and is prone to bully other children. In both of these last cases the child's behaviour is likely to elicit an unfavourable response from the parent so that vicious circles develop...as a child grows older, the pattern becomes increasingly a property of the child himself, which means that he tends to impose it, or some derivative of it, upon new relationships such as with a teacher, a foster-parent or a therapist...once built, evidence suggests, these models of a parent and self in interaction tend to persist and are so taken for granted that they come to operate at an unconscious level. (pp.126–7, p.130)

When people develop a dementing illness and are in need of services, the personality that they bring with them is the end result of years of development, and may be considerably damaged in a number of areas. Service providers may be completely unaware of what caused the damage and, of course, it will have nothing to do with their present illness. However, their ability to cope with their illness, to cope with meeting new people and new situations, and to 'live with themselves' will have been developed over the years. As Cotrell and Lein (1993) observed:

> behaviour observed...may have antecedents in the victim's less impaired history...by introducing a psychosocial perspective into what has been predominantly a biomedical experience, we may be able to identify factors that hinder or enhance the successful

adaptation of the individual to the dementing illness...indeed, we may find that much of the variability in the progression of the disease can be accounted for by psychosocial differences. The benefits of such knowledge include an enhanced quality of life for the dementia victim and fewer problem behaviours and psychiatric symptoms to be managed by the caregiver. (p.128)

Cotrell and Lein interpret behavioural disturbances as adaptive attempts by the individual, often in collusion with the caregiver, to avoid confrontation with the reality of existing intellectual deficits. I shall be looking at problem behaviours in greater detail in Chapter 11.

The death of a parent has been the subject of work done in Holland on the phenomenon of parent-fixation in some elderly people with dementia. Meisen has argued that parent-fixation is a key to unlocking the experiential world of elderly people with dementia in which feelings of unsafety trigger attachment behaviours. This has been discussed in an article by Marie Mills (1992). Writing about the importance of memories in general she points out that they help us to perceive ourselves as unique individuals with our own particular experiences, and the recalling of past memories enables the person with dementia to remember, even for a short period of time, the person that they once were. But it can be a skilled job handling memories, as one support worker commented:

> I agree with life stories as the basis for communication and as a guide to the type of service we offer that person although I have experienced a few situations where the life story has been too distressing for the individual to cope with and has resulted in anger, anxiety, mild depression for that individual. This is quite damaging for the client especially if they cannot be helped by untrained care staff who do not know how to respond appropriately.

As Mills (1992) reflected

> it is possible that some of the strong emotions expressed by the elderly people during these interviews could have been overwhelming for someone without some knowledge of counselling strategies...it is a natural defence to 'block' or deny strong feelings in other people if the recipient feels unable, or inadequate to cope with them. This can be standard practice in the nursing milieu due to lack of training in counselling techniques and the pressure of work...counselling skills would enable the nurse/carer and demented person to converse in a more socially interactive manner. (p.9)

Conclusion

It seems abundantly clear from all the replies that I received that if we are to individualise care for people, then knowing about them, their life story, their achievements, their experiences (good or bad) and their likes and dislikes is of enormous importance. However, it is one thing to accept that this is important and it is quite another matter to ensure that structures are set up in such a way as to enable staff to have both the time and the skills to engage in this sort of work. It is also clear that a great many people with dementia are able to share in this activity and communicate to those who are exploring the past with them. As so often seems to be the case, there is very much more that people with dementia are able to communicate than most services and service providers seem to be willing to accept. If we have the desire, the determination, the skills and the time then the process of communication can be considerably eased if we follow the route of discovering more about the person's past.

CHAPTER 9

The Effect of the Environment

> *This chapter sets communication in the widest of contexts, arguing that design, space, light, colour and noise can all have considerable effect upon people's ability to communicate with each other. The time of day, the physical location and the relationship between the people communicating can all have an effect upon the effectiveness of that process. Thus we need to have an awareness of the possible influence of external environmental factors before we make any kind of judgment on people's ability to communicate.*

Alan Dunlop (1994), in an excellent literature review on designing environments for people with dementia, writes:

> The 'Environmental Docility Hypothesis' performed by Lawton and Nahemow (1973) contends that 'limitations in health, cognitive skills, ego strength, status, social role performance or degree of cultural evolution will tend to heighten the docility of the person in the face of environmental constraints and influences'. Once we wade through the jargon and tortuous language we find that the hypothesis once again supports the premise that the physical environment can influence the behaviour of people who have cognitive impairment. (p.3)

I was interested to explore whether the environment in which people lived had much effect upon their ability to communicate. In my consultative document I suggested that

> the ability of a person with dementia to communicate was influenced by such factors as location, the time of day, background noises, colour, the intensity of lighting and general fatigue. It also seems to be related

to the nature of the relationship that the person has with whoever is providing the service or is talking with them.

I then asked whether people had any experience of changes taking place when any of these variables changed. The response was overwhelmingly supportive of the view that I put forward. I am taking a very wide view of environmental factors in this chapter. It can be argued that they are very much secondary in the communicative process, but I am of the opinion that providing an appropriate milieu is an important ingredient in the mixture of factors which combine to produce the possibilities for effective communication.

The proprietor of a residential home commented that

> loud, brash, intense colour or music often frighten and threaten people with dementia…decor can be subdued, colour splashes coming from things chosen jointly, such as pictures, flowers, ornaments…suitable music, approaching people quietly and calmly, speaking and touching gently. Change in floor covering can be very disorienting…some will be unwilling to step from one to the other.

A principal officer for the elderly and physically disabled had much to say about this subject:

> I am very concerned about how units for people with dementia are built. There has to be a way of 'signposting' inside the building and very often numbering or naming rooms has no meaning whatsoever for the person with dementia. Colour co-ordination may be helpful here, but also I am thinking about the layout of the bedrooms and communal areas. In one's own home one doesn't walk the length of a very long corridor to get to a place where one can socialise. As indeed it is very important to have a quiet and peaceful regime when one goes to bed. In one's own home you don't actually have twenty other people downstairs in your living room while you are going up to bed, with all the attendant noise. Bedtime should be an extremely peaceful time of the day and, in my experience in many residential homes, this is the noisiest time of the day. Background noise is very important – we have no way of knowing what effect noise can have on a person with dementia. One of the reasons why they become extremely disturbed and start to scream and shout is because they are trying to overcome the awful 'white' noise to which they are subjected. I am thinking in particular of very loud TV sets in communal lounges. I feel that the layout of gardens in residential homes should be carefully looked at. There should be access to gardens where a person can possibly enjoy just looking at plants and flowers, or possibly being

able to do a bit of gardening. I do not subscribe to the theory of 'wandering'; in my experience people with dementia do not wander, they are actually setting out to go somewhere with a purpose. It is understanding what that purpose is that is the challenge. Also it is not always fully acknowledged that they have likes and dislikes, as we all do, and there may be people with whom they get on very well and others to whom they take an intense dislike. It is important therefore to understand the feelings that come into play with personal interaction.

Some of these concerns were echoed in remarks made by a clinical neuro-psychologist:

> In my last place of work I would walk onto the dementia care ward and find the lights turned off and the radio on. Sometimes the sun was shining outside so it was gloomy by comparison inside; sometimes the television was competing with the radio. Almost inevitably I would turn on the lights and, if no one was listening to the radio, turn it or the television off. When asking the reason for this, the reply was that keeping the room darker kept the patients quieter and that they enjoyed the radio! I was never convinced about either argument. These seemed to me to be highly manipulative actions on the part of the staff. I play the radio when I want to listen to something. It is not too difficult to ask someone with dementia if they would like to listen to some music or watch a programme. By establishing their preferences in advance a choice could be made about what to listen to…if no one is listening then it should stay off as it only adds to the difficulty of filtering stimuli. Despite the fact that we know how much more effective communication with people with dementia is if environmental noise and distraction is kept to a minimum, many so-called specialist wards are confusing places to be.

A senior occupational therapist, working in the area of elderly mental health, was quite sure that environmental factors were important. She said that it was 'essential' to consider them when planning a group, and she commented how she used the physical characteristics of her workroom to assist her.

> The OT [Occupational Therapy] room used for groups is a separate room opposite the clients' day room on the ward, with a large window overlooking the entrance to the unit. Clients appear to enjoy looking out of the window as they can actually see cars and people coming and going, and also observe the weather and the seasons. Giving people the opportunity to watch outside activity is often enough to

spark conversation without any prompting from the staff, and at times an organised activity is not necessary.

I also find that clients appear to enjoy coming into the OT room as it has a very different feel to it than the rest of the ward – it is very quiet and feels separate from the noise and activity of the rest of the ward.

With groups we have found that 'active' groups (exercise, cooking, art) are more appropriate to run in the morning, and groups which are 'social' or 'talking' often work better in the early afternoon…it is essential to have a flexible approach when running groups and spend a lot of time planning a session or activity – using the right room, chairs, tables etc.…seating in an activity is important. I have found it easier to focus people on a task if they are sitting on upright dining chairs with a table in front of them…if clients are sitting in armchairs with no table, it is much harder for them to focus on the activity… I have also found that individuals interact with other group members if they are sitting around a table.

The co-ordinator of a day care centre commented that:

> the nature of relationships is most important here. The physical environment is secondary, but must be warm and bright. It can be too warm and too tranquil and induce sleep (see many residential and nursing homes!). A change of leader or change of venue can have marked effects. Background noise, and over-bright lights etc. prevent communication and concentration. Background music we find is not a good idea. Attention to making a person *physically* comfortable must improve the ability to communicate. We find it almost impossible to get certain things dealt with, for example – painful feet, inadequate hearing aids, ill-fitting dentures and ill-fitting spectacles. It appears to be so much easier for a person with dementia to be provided with a nice deep armchair (difficult to get out of?) than for these factors to be dealt with. I suggest that we would all lapse into inertia if we had to endure some or all of these things – or become aggressive.

Another occupational therapist said that she

> had experience of many clients being at their best in the late morning and early evening. Also, colour of decor – light green works well in 'soothing' distressed and aggressive clients. Our OT department is designed with this in mind. We try to meet clients where there is *no* background noise.

The importance of these things was stressed by a consultant physician in elderly medicine who wrote:

> I would entirely agree that environmental factors affect both behaviour and communication. There has been relatively little systematic study of this area and this is urgently needed. This should facilitate behavioural approaches to patients and decrease the amount of drug prescription.

The time of day

Many of the respondents commented that people react differently to different things and different people at different times of the day. Therefore, it is not possible to know what a person is capable of understanding, or how easy it is to communicate with them unless we have seen them at different times of the day, over a period of time. Someone who is very 'distant' and difficult to communicate with in the morning may be very much more approachable in the afternoon, for instance. As one carer wrote, 'visits should be made at different times of the day and one will soon learn the best time to visit and have a reasonable conversation'. A social worker made the same point, saying:

> I have noticed that the time of day can make a large difference – it is useful for [service] providers to meet the person at different times of the day to see whether this makes a difference.

A development officer commented that

> the time of day has a profound effect on some people, particularly when winter and the darker nights are concerned. Some become more restless as it grows darker and want to get home. Fatigue also links into this where people become more tired by the end of the day and this can influence behaviour (increased confusion/distress/lack of 'coping' with information etc.).

The manager of a day care centre commented:

> I have always found that communication is always better in the early part of the day when the atmosphere is quiet, relaxed and warm and people's basic needs are met. Should the noise level increase in whatever area then the level of agitation increases and any communication beyond superficial level is almost impossible.

Noise

Many people commented upon the problems posed by noise, and several of the earlier quotations mentioned noise whilst making a comment about a different factor. The noise from radios and televisions seems to be an almost universal feature of residential care, and I can vividly remember how difficult I found it to talk to a colleague in one particular establishment because of the volume of the radio. Not only was no one paying any attention to it, it was also proving to be an effective discouragement to conversation even to those who wanted to speak! In many places there seems to be an almost irresistible urge to have the radio and the television competing with each other.

The sister/manager of a day care centre wrote:

> background noise is a definite irritant. Vacuum cleaning at our centre in the main lounge is normally done after members have gone home. A workman putting in airbricks outside the building caused a lot of irritation, particularly amongst the men. The centre staff also found it irksome! Music too loud causes annoyance. We have a gentleman who sings out of tune and ahead of everyone else, so a member of staff now takes him to another room to sing, thus allowing the other members to enjoy the pianist and their sing-along.

A respondent who works on dementia care mapping commented that

> noise is without doubt a negative factor in both concentration and emotional well-being. I find it significant that so many people involved in caring for people with dementia say that sufferers 'do not know what is happening to them – it's a blessing really'. This seems to serve two purposes – firstly, they do not have to care so much with the environment (physical and social) that they provide and, second, they are shielded from the pain of realising that people with dementia *do* know what is happening to them and just how frightening a prospect that is. Once we can take this on board, we can start furnishing the context of care with the warmth and peace and companionship which facilitate good communication with anyone.

Location

One of the most telling remarks that emerged during the whole of this project came from a project manager in priority services, who wrote:

> This might seem a daft thing to say but is it not common sense to assume that by removing someone from their own home and placing

them in a strange ward, full of strange people and routines, [and] to assess their level of confusion, you will discover a very very confused person?

Where a person is seen seems to have quite a marked effect on their ability to communicate. A senior physiotherapist remarked that she

> had worked in hospital and community settings and, particularly in hospital, there can be a good deal of background noise which interferes with good communication. In such a situation, with others around to listen, it is also not always relaxing for the client. We often used to treat people in the physio department for one session (even if they didn't need to be seen off the ward), just to see if communication was easier – it often was. Also in ward settings, with people who have difficulty concentrating, there are a lot of potential distractions and interruptions.

In the community, I have found that people are generally more relaxed in their own homes. The only exception is when there is a client/carer conflict which can strongly prejudice the outcome of our assessment of the situation if we are not extremely objective.

A social work team leader stressed the importance of recognising the effect of location and commented that the setting in which the interview takes place can be 'critical in terms of determining the outcome'.

Several people commented on the differences that can occur in behaviour and in communication by taking a person outside and walking or talking with them away from the distractions that so often confuse people inside lounges or in rooms where there are other people. A charge nurse in an elderly mentally infirm acute/assessment ward wrote:

> in my experience, simply taking someone out into the fresh air can effect a big change in responses and behaviour, thus affecting communication in a positive way.

The weather also, it seems, can have an effect upon people's communicative abilities. One person commented:

> it would appear to me that all the factors identified play a part in determining the effectiveness or otherwise of communication. The weather is another factor – 'I'm feeling very disturbed today. The wind is definitely getting up. Can you see the way it throws about the trees and things?'.

The Social Services Inspectorate Report (1993) *Inspecting for Quality* highlighted the problem of location indicators when it said:

> Modern logos such as matchstick men and women, to identify toilet
> areas, may not always be comprehensible to this generation of elderly
> people with mental disorders and other cues may be necessary...
> Equally, furniture of uniform design and finish may be aesthetically
> pleasing but it is unlikely to help identify location for people with
> cognitive impairment. (p.20)

Light

A piece of research (Ford *et al.* 1986) was carried out in the mid 1980s to
monitor the effect of changing the environment for people with dementia
in terms of lighting and background music. Nursing staff became interested
in the possibilities of this research when they noted that patients became
calmer during a power failure resulting from a mid-afternoon thunderstorm;
they had also noticed that patients often raised their feet much higher when
walking through doorways made with darker tiles. The researchers noted
that in treatment settings it had been reported that the use of bright, artificial
lighting had significantly influenced depressive symptoms in manic depres-
sives, and they knew that the use of bright colours and signposts as
orientation aides for confused people had been found to be helpful; so they
asked the question 'What effects do the environmental stimuli of light and
sound have on the confused, agitated behaviour of patients with Alzheimer's
disease?'

What they found was that by lowering the lighting level during meal
times, all the patients demonstrated a decrease in disturbed behaviour and a
return to increased intensity and frequency when florescent light was
reintroduced. The staff reported that there was an increase in food consump-
tion and a 50 per cent decrease in the length of time that the meal took
when the low lighting was introduced, and the noise level decreased. They
also reported that they themselves also felt calmer.

The effect of music on patient agitation was more complex to analyse.
The noise level overall was lower with white music than without, but not as
low as when the lighting was reduced. They then introduced Country and
Western music ('selected because of its familiarity to patients in the ward')
and this resulted in increased frequency and duration of all the behaviours
they had previously identified as being problematic. They also played a tape
of nature sounds and soothing music and this resulted in a decreased noise
level. It also decreased the 'verbal criterion levels in all but one patient who
moaned almost continuously and one patient who whistled with a bird song'.

A few people responding to the consultative document commented on lighting, but not in such a way as to enable me to make any conclusions. A nurse manager reported that changing the ward lighting from overhead lights to wall lights had helped considerably, whilst someone else observed that one ward had introduced softer lighting at meal times 'and it has been noticed that the clients are calmer, especially at the 6pm supper'. Another comment on lighting came from a charge nurse who said that dim lights in toilets in a new building had caused people to disorientate and increasing the intensity of the lighting had improved matters.

Colour

Not a great deal is known about the effect of colour on people with dementia, but there is a growing awareness that different colours might increase or decrease confusion, and that they might also convey 'hidden messages'. One person wrote in giving an example of the effect of colour:

> a lady showing signs of acute dementia in a residential home had her bedroom redecorated and the colour scheme was mauve and purple – curtains, bedspread, wallpaper etc. It looked extremely nice but the lady could not go into the room without becoming extremely distressed and it became so bad she became almost hysterical. It was later discovered that there was very scant information about her past, but she had in fact been brought up a very strict Roman Catholic and associated mauve and purple with mourning and death. Her association with the colour of the room was that she would almost certainly die in there. When her room was changed to another part of the building there were no problems and no more distress.

Alan Dunlop (1994) cites a dementia unit in Northern Ireland at which a test was carried out to judge the ability of people with dementia to recognise colour. This showed that the majority of residents were able to identify and recognise different colours and consequently – after further tests to establish preferences and the ability to distinguish certain colours more easily than others – toilet doors were painted pink and bedroom doors were painted peach.

> Since the scheme's inception staff have reported a decrease in behavioural disturbances and aggressive outbursts among residents and the scheme also proved less burdensome to the staff who now spend less time escorting residents to the toilet. (pp.6–7)

Further work done on colour has been described by Bell (1992), and Mary Kelly (1993) refers to how colour might be used when considering other factors:

> It cannot be overstated that the number of doors should be kept to an absolute minimum, particularly where they open off a circulation route. Where doors cannot be avoided they should be treated according to their relevance to the residents. Relevant doors, i.e. those to toilets, should be highlighted through the use of colour, signs and symbols. Bedroom doors can be denoted through the use of pictures, colours, signs etc. clearly showing the use of the rooms behind the doors. (p.9)

The Social Services Inspectorate Report (1993) commented that there was evidence to suggest that

> wallpaper with complicated patterns may have a negative effect and that soft pastel colours which tone into each other may make it more difficult for people with cognitive difficulties to find their way around, to identify doors in walls or to identify where they are in a building. Similarly, floor coverings with strong colour contrasts in their patterns as one moves from room to room may be perceived as changes of floor level by some people. (p.20)

Space

A director of clinical development wrote about the use of space:

> The use of space sets the scene in which the person trying to cope with their illness can be either constructive or destructive. By planning an environment which is comfortable and stimulating, which promotes a sense of freedom whilst acknowledging safety aspects, the person can feel 'at home' in hospital.

The issue of corridors is one of considerable controversy. Some people say that it is good to have passageways in which people can walk to their heart's content, whilst others claim that they add to confusion and agitation. Milke (1992) writing from Canada says that

> wandering pathways have become a standard design recommendation for special care units and other facilities that care for people with dementia...the shape of a pathway is often prescribed e.g. 'The preferred approach is a layout, such as a loop or a figure eight, in

which the pacer never comes to a dead end'…one dementia ward has considered purchasing a treadmill. (p.133)

She goes on to comment that it is important to note that there have been no adequate evaluations of the loops, ovals and figure of eight configurations that many people advocate. She also suggests that much walking is actually influenced by the physical environment and that providing long walkways encouraged people to walk.

Milke quotes the ideas of Spivack (1967), who suggests that 'a corridor becomes unpleasant when it has five or more equally spaced doors down one side, and when it is five times as long as its width', and she quotes work by Beattie (1974) who claimed that visual hazards were caused by:

- excessive length (anything beyond the distance limits for being able to see faces and facial expressions)
- illusions of endless space
- multiple choice points
- disturbing surface patterns, such as repetitive lines or chessboard squares.

She said that it has been shown that the ability of a person to see their goal or desired location from their present position significantly increases their ability to move independently, and therefore contributes to their self-sufficiency and sense of well-being.

Other factors

Noni Cobban (1994) has written an informative and interesting paper on carpets in which she discusses the pros and cons of carpets versus linoleum and vinyl. She says that the control of odour is not the only reason for choosing one type of flooring rather than another, and she discusses appearance, warmth, maintenance, cleaning, safety, quietness and many other aspects which need to be taken into consideration when making a choice about floor covering. These, in themselves, may not have a direct influence upon facilitating communication, but they are important in the general well-being of people with dementia, and therefore have a knock-on effect as far as communication is concerned.

She says that she has no doubts that the surroundings in which a person lives have an effect upon the attitude of those coming into contact with them, and closes her paper with the following story.

> The first time I met this lady was in response to a call from her emergency alarm early one morning. When I arrived at her house, I found that she had fallen, had been incontinent and was half-dressed in rather stained clothes. The house was run down, cold and dingy, and not very clean, and, after attending to her and leaving her with a cup of tea, I found myself questioning the quality of this lady's life, thinking that she may be more comfortable in a nursing home. A few weeks later I was called to her house again and was pleasantly surprised to see that it had been redecorated and carpeted, and a new heater had been installed. She was cheerful and obviously happy. Again, the improved surroundings had affected my perception of her and her situation. (p.6)

It seems probable that it was not only the writer's perceptions that had been altered by the changed environment, but also the lady's sense of well-being and independence.

A unit manager wrote in, agreeing with the importance of environmental influences, but also stressing that continuity and stability were also important and that 'if the variables change it can be very unnerving for the person with dementia. For example, day centres closing on a bank holiday can alter the routine of the person, resulting in uncertainty about the day, time and place'.

Several people commented on the desirability of having a stimulating environment, and this was summed up by comments from a project manager whose father had dementia.

> I noticed his condition deteriorated markedly in a relatively short space of time when he went into residential care. I believe his deterioration may have been due to lack of one to one attention and stimulation generally... There was absolutely no stimulation in the long-stay hospital ward where he was ultimately transferred. Patients were left to sit or wander around the ward and no effort was made to have any form of activity.

Whilst another respondent wrote that:

> my mother is more responsive since father took up residence in the same nursing home and is able to spend more time with her and help her with each meal.

Relationships are not part of the physical environment, but they are part of the total environment and it is clear that communication is greatly eased if there is a trusting, stable relationship providing the context within which it takes place. It was pointed out that 'the nature of the relationship is very important. If the patient dislikes the person he will ignore their attempts to communicate'.

A clinical nurse specialist noticed

> major changes when we changed from single sex facility to mixed – there was a general improvement in behaviour. Also a move from a busy 'corridor ward' to a quieter facility showed improved behaviour of residents. Patient communication was enhanced by the staff speaking quietly.

And the obvious was stated by an Inspector – or perhaps it is not so obvious in some places:

> There is the need to recognise that some simple care tasks, such as ensuring that spectacles are clean, appropriate for the user and worn; and that hearing aids are clean, in working order and worn, are an aid to communication... I have visited a residential home recently where the clock in the lounge is always wrong and there are significant difficulties in communicating with at least one resident about which meal is next in the day.

A development nurse sent in the following scenario, which, with variations, could no doubt be echoed by many people. Commenting on the suggestion that people's abilities to communicate are affected by external environmental factors she wrote:

> I wholeheartedly agree. However the reality in many areas of care for people with dementia is rather far removed from this. Our ward is located in a very old building that hundreds of years ago used to be a French prisoner of war base. Following that it became a local workhouse and then it was converted to a hospital for the elderly. The very impressive but formidable building next door was originally a lunatic asylum where unfortunate people from the workhouse would be sent 'for their sins', and until a few years ago remained the local psychiatric hospital. Since then there has been a retrenchment that amalgamated Mental Health Services with the Elderly Care Department on our site, but a new Regional Secure Unit has been established on the fringes of these grounds. Predictably we are separated from the main general hospital site and are on the fringes of the city, so it is not difficult to imagine the extent of the very negative image we have inherited, both among the local population and other health care professionals in the Trust. It is extremely difficult to turn this stereotyping around despite the developments and

foresight of many people working here. Our local elderly beg not to be sent here from the admission ward on the main hospital site, while confused elderly patients often ask what they have done wrong in being 'sent' here. Notwithstanding the implications of the dementing process which already undermines them, this becomes an additional barrier to promoting a feeling of well-being.

Reflection

It seems quite clear that the ability of many people with dementia to communicate is considerably influenced by a whole number of external environmental factors. Change the environment and some people are more able – or less able – to communicate. So when making any judgment about a person's communicative abilities, such judgment needs to be set within an awareness of the total environment of that person.

Most of the illustrations given above come from different types of residential placement, but we know that majority of people with dementia are looked after in their local community. They live alone or with their partner, and are cared for by family, neighbours and friends. It is estimated that in Scotland by the year 2013 there will be some 116,000 people with dementia, of whom 94,000 will live at home (Burley and Pollock 1992). It is therefore essential that we find ways of translating what we know about environmental influences in residential settings into domestic settings. As Burley and Pollock argue:

> If we accept that elderly people would prefer to stay in their own home and that their carers, in the main, also prefer to maintain their relatives at home, we can expect that during the next decade about four out of five people with dementia will continue to be living at home. This being the case should we not be doing far more to organise and plan the house and its environment to be more comprehensible to people who suffer from disorientation? (p.2)

All buildings have characteristics which either assist or hinder people with dementia. The more sensitive we are to such characteristics, the more likely it will be that the person with dementia will be assisted. The more relaxed and secure the person feels, the more likely it will be that he or she is able to communicate.

CHAPTER 10

Nonverbal Communication

People can communicate in many different ways and not all of them require speech. It is probable that many opportunities are missed because carers are not sufficiently skilled in recognising and interpreting nonverbal communication. Touch is of enormous importance, ranging from holding a person's hand to formal massage. Music, art and aromatherapy are all being used in some establishments. Whilst many people recognise the value of nonverbal communication, there is little evidence to suggest that it is widely promoted or encouraged in dementia care, and there were many requests for further training in this area.

> There are, in fact, no more important communications between one human being and another than those expressed emotionally, and no information more vital for constructing and reconstructing working models of self and other than information about how each feels toward the other. (Bowlby 1988, p.156)

There are many ways in which people communicate, and speech is not an essential requirement of them all. It may be possible for people to express their preferences or their feelings even though they have difficulties in communicating by speech. In my consultative document I suggested that

> many people gain insight into the views and preferences, the mood and sense of well-being of people with dementia through art, music and different forms of touch.

I put forward the view that people who find verbal expression difficult invariably find other ways in which to communicate. I then asked people what their experience of nonverbal communication was and whether they thought that such an approach might be able to enrich their work. Of all the subjects raised in the consultative document, this is the one which people responded to most by way of asking for further information and training. It seems obvious that if people cannot communicate by word of mouth then they might find other ways, but it would appear that an awareness of this is often neglected in dementia care.

Tom Kitwood (1993b) has commented that

> dementia sufferers sometimes seem to have a heightened awareness of body language, and often their main meanings may be conveyed nonverbally. In the case of those who are very severely impaired in cognition, it seems probable that the words and sentences are at times more of an accompaniment or adornment than the vehicle for carrying the significant message... (p.64)

> ...the theory sheds new light on why dementia care, whether in family or in institutional settings, has often failed. So many gestures have passed unnoticed, or been ignored or discounted; so many communicative acts have been aborted; so many gross impositions have been made upon the dementia sufferer from others' frame of reference. The hope for dementia care, within new patterns that are currently being created, is that a far higher level of communicative competence may be possible than has actually been believed. The key concepts here are 'holding' and 'facilitation'. Although all this may appear to make extra demands upon the caregiver, the general experience seems to be that the kind of approach I have described here makes care work less exhausting; it can even, at times, be stimulating and refreshing'. (p.65)

The proprietor of a residential home shared her experiences:

> I find that nonverbal communication is often preferred by people with dementia even when they can communicate verbally...the most important form of communication is tactile. When speaking, we touch residents, kiss them goodnight, hello and goodbye – our residents respond in kind – through this, their mood, wants and needs can be interpreted. Staff have become very skilled at this – we also have a dog and two cats, we find that they are the single most important factor in helping new residents to settle down.

A development nurse in dementia services commented that many of the people that she worked with communicated their frustration very effectively through challenging behaviour, but added that persuading professionals to see it that way cannot be done quite so easily. Persuading them to identify nonverbal distress before it becomes challenging behaviour is even more difficult. To take the issue of nonverbal communication a little further, I believe that people with dementia become extremely astute at reading our body language. They often fail to understand our 'language' or what we want them to do but even though our words are often meaningless to them they are able to establish a lot of what we want through our nonverbals. If the carers of people with this disease became half as effective at reading body language as the sufferers, we would be significantly more advanced in our attempts to communicate with them.

A consultant clinical psychologist observed that

> therapies such as the approach of Validation Therapy places great emphasis on nonverbal aspects of communication, and their use in building rapport with people with dementia – for example with breathing and posture. Within our service we have also been exploring the value of complementary therapies including aromatherapy, in relieving distress and promoting well-being.

The importance of touch

A number of people wrote in discussing alternative therapies and approaches, and some of these will be considered later. The vast majority of people stressed the importance of touch, and the need to be sensitive, and aware of the need of many people to hold and be held. A sample of the comments is given here:

- In my experience, cuddling my father or holding his hand is a great means of making him feel happy.
- Touch is very important and validating…often people with dementia have reduced networks and changing relationships and therefore do not have the same positive experiences of touching that we may be accustomed to. I am always very struck by the notion that some people may only be touched when they are having something done to them – this cannot be said to be a validating experience.
- Touch becomes very important – reassurance by stroking or holding hands can be more effective than verbal communication.
- Touch is of great value – more so the elderly who may have lost their partner and are starved of the warm physical relationship which has been part of their lives for so long – hand and foot massage is a

good way of touching that can be physically as well as emotionally therapeutic.

○ I find my mother brighter-eyed and smiling and [she] appears more content when physical contact is made either by touching her hands or giving a kiss on her cheek or even when her face is massaged.

○ Hand massage was introduced by the occupational therapists and is carried on by the nurses. Many patients enjoy physical contact. Foot massage and aromatherapy are also being introduced.

○ I find that touch is a critical factor. I can communicate a great deal by the way that I hold a person's hand. And I believe I can tell a great deal about their emotional state by the pressure exerted in return. Eye contact, tone of voice and body posture are also key components of communication with people with dementia.

A specialist in old age psychiatry confessed that 'this is not an area I recall ever having been discussed amongst my colleagues – perhaps putting it on the agenda might be a good way to start!', and went on to say:

> physical contact often seems to play a major part in my contact with people who are severely impaired – hugging, stroking, holding hands. I am not wholly clear in my mind whose needs are best met by actions of this kind. When words have failed it feel like the only potent way of expressing support, and that one is concerned.

There can be dangers in touching, of course, and we need to be careful that such actions are appropriate to the person and to the situation. Not everyone wants to establish contact with people in this way, and carers must be vigilant not to abuse the relationships of trust that many people with dementia build up with them. There can also be a difference between touch and communication, they are not necessarily the same thing. We are accepting the importance of touch, but there needs to be a lot of thought given to how we communicate by touch. Even more thought needs to be given to how we interpret the responses to our touches, and what we are meaning to communicate by them in the first place. It was this area which prompted so many requests for training and elaboration.

The importance of touch was explored in an article by Lennie Seaman (1982) who commented that if a nurse touches a patient when no task is involved, he/she is clearly saying 'I don't have to touch you, but I want to', and such touching is a powerful therapeutic intervention. The elderly probably have a greater need for meaningful touch because of decreasing visual, hearing and functional capabilities which limit their experiential capacity. The lack of meaningful touch can therefore make their sense of isolation even greater. Seaman (1982) notes that:

> the infant explores the world through touch. The child cannot solve problems but learns by the repetition of actions reinforced by reward and punishment. Many of the early conditioned responses are learned at nonverbal level and seem to persist in advanced age, even in the presence of brain damage...due to the conditioning nature of early learning, nonverbal language takes on particular importance with confused patients in situations where words fail completely. Consequently, nonverbal communication, such as touch, may be successful when neural pathology prevents comprehension of verbal communication...unless repeated contact through touch is made with regressed patients, they will withdraw. And if there is an inability to speak, the isolation is even more profound. Because nonverbal communication appears to be retained in the confused person after more complex behaviours no longer exist, nurses can endeavour to maintain contact with the confused, regressed patient through frequent affective touch. (p.163)

The staff nurse in a nursing home recounted the story of how touch enabled a process of communication to unfold:

> One elderly lady who liked massage and had her own masseuse each month used to allow me to massage her feet and the fragile shins of her legs. She had Parkinson's disease and had been a biochemist. One day she abstractly said to me 'the quality of mercy...' I had learned this from Portia's speech in *The Merchant of Venice* when I was thirteen years old, and so I continued it for her – and we said it together many times until she died. 'The quality of mercy is not strained. It droppeth as the gentle rain from heaven upon the earth beneath, 'tis twice blessed. It blesseth him who gives and him who takes.'... Patience and trust, love and deep understanding can give much to these people and it is an aspect of my work which I find deeply satisfying.

Music

I have heard of the work of a music therapist who enabled people to express their emotions by the way in which they played various percussion instruments, and by a careful selection of music he was able to mirror the various moods of people, and enabled them to 'own' feelings that had been repressed. Various people wrote in sharing their experiences with music, such as this contribution from a senior occupational therapist in the area of elderly mental health:

> I have one client, in her early sixties and with a very advanced condition. She has no speech and is very restless, usually pacing the corridors for much of the day, and it can be very difficult to get her to sit down and rest or eat a meal etc. Initially I felt at a loss when trying to think of an activity which she could join in with. Painting was tried, as she had previously enjoyed this, but she remained very restless and had great difficulty handling a brush or using it purposefully. She was then tried in a music group where clients were given a choice of music and the opportunity to sit and listen. The change in her behaviour was marked. She was able to sit for at least an hour, showing no signs of restlessness. From her expression, she appeared very calm and relaxed and content, and at times tapped her foot or her fingers to the music. We will be going on to try letting her listen to music prior to an activity (such as lunch) to see if it makes her less restless and easier to feed. In an ideal work place, staff would look for key nonverbal forms of communication, but unfortunately this is very time-consuming – in regard to the occupational therapy service there are ninety clients and three staff, so we cannot be involved with everyone.

A nursing sister explained how difficult it was to convince other staff that this sort of approach was important:

> mood and emotional state is often communicated more easily in non-verbal ways. In an attempt to create an environment which respects the need for different forms of communication we are finding that many people (staff) have negative attitudes towards music, dance, art, drama etc. It is often perceived as being a bit 'fairy' and not essential to care. A lot of education is needed before these types of attitudes will alter.

Aromatherapy

Quite a number of people mentioned that they were exploring aromatherapy as a way of communicating with people in more advanced stages of dementia. It serves to calm people and encourages relaxation and a sense of well-being. A deputy manager in a home for older people wrote that:

> a student is preparing to do some reminiscence work on smells with a group of three residents whose verbal expression is significantly impaired. This area is very exciting, but I feel that local authority

homes are disadvantaged. We pay our staff well and consequently have good staff who are well capable of doing innovative work, but we have neither the staffing levels within our homes nor the finances to purchase outside services to develop this kind of thing.

Art and drama

A most attractively produced book *Memories in the Making* (Jenny 1994) contains a selection of paintings produced by people with Alzheimer's disease in California. The workshops which produced these pictures are run on the assumption that

> the patient has many things they would like to say and there is some meaning in what these people say or do, no matter how garbled their verbal expression might be. It also assumes that they can do more than they have been given credit for to date. (p.3)

As one of the artists said 'It feels so good when people listen to you sometimes instead of them telling you to do so much – so much – so much…'

One lady I visited spent much of the day painting. She came alive when she showed me her pictures, which were pinned all over the walls of the house. She found a sense of self-worth in her art, and discovered that other people were interested in both her pictures and herself. Several people wrote about the value of art, but most of the comments were extremely tentative, and were usually coupled with requests for guidance and better resources. Typical was the comment from a clinical services manager:

> Art and music therapy should be readily available to people with dementia. This is an area that requires further development and resources.

A sector manager wrote that she had found

> the use of music therapy, art therapy and drama therapy extremely effective in stimulating interest and in opening up channels of communication. In working with a drama therapist and a small group, many of whom had not spoken or made contact with others for some time, we mimed old tasks such as washing clothes, cooking etc., and the response was astonishing. To use such techniques in local authority settings requires extra funding from outside sources, something we have only achieved short term in our authority. It is always seen as a 'luxury' when service provision is being cut all around us.

Paula Crimmens (1994) gave a fascinating talk on drama therapy at an international conference on Alzheimer's disease:

> one of the things we worked really hard to create and reinforce with virtually everything we did was the opportunity for people to be individuals with their needs and preferences respected, and still be valued members of the group. This meant that we did not seduce, cajole or bully anyone into doing something they didn't want to and instead always offered them choice and initiative. Offering choice and initiative is a major theme in Drama therapy...a common misconception is that the elderly person who is dementing cannot make a choice. I work on the belief that they can and it is up to me to take the time to interpret that person's wishes as accurately and as sensitively as I can...our principal aim behind every session is to create opportunities for contact...contact is about person to person as opposed to role to role. It is genuine, open and reciprocated. Contact is the road to intimacy. It can take many forms – verbal, nonverbal, body language... (p.3)

Conclusion

A telling comment came from a social work teacher and researcher:

> While I am sure that nonverbal communication is exceedingly important, it would be a shame to let ourselves off too lightly in trying also to develop our skills in effective verbal communication. Perhaps if we became more skilled in lessening the sense of threat, people with dementia would need to retreat less into either symbolic or nonverbal communication. Improved communication, to some extent, would follow on from a sense of improved well-being and security. This would need to be reinforced by explicit demonstration of our willingness and ability to share the world of the person with dementia and attend to the things which are important to them within their time-scale. I think there are no shortcuts. It takes time and a capacity not to be overwhelmingly frightened by the fearfulness of the other's pain. [We need] some illustrative teaching tapes of examples of verbal and nonverbal communicating with people with dementia as often, I suspect, workers ignore even basic skills such as stage setting, positioning, pacing, voice modulation, rephrasing and structuring of content, let alone the more sophisticated skills.

The need for training was the predominant message that came from the responses to my consultative document. There seemed to be a general agreement that people can communicate nonverbally, but the illustrations and examples of how this was achieved or understood were fairly sparse. There was a general understanding of the value and importance of touch, and this is obviously an area that is being developed, with more and more services incorporating massage, both formal and informal. There was often the sense of this being a relatively recent discovery, and one suspects that the number of places where touch is seen as an essential element of care, and where it is talked about and evaluated and actively promoted, is still in a small minority. Even where there was a knowledge of the importance of music, art and drama, this seldom seemed to have been taken up and analysed. It tended to be seen as a pleasurable pastime and an activity through which some people were able to express themselves more easily. It was seen to be a costly addition to basic care and one which few establishments had the necessary resources to allocate to it. All in all, despite an awareness that people can communicate nonverbally, there were few examples of sustained work being done to interpret the nonverbal language of people with dementia.

CHAPTER 11

Challenging Behaviour

Dementia does not only affect the mind. For a great many people it also has an effect upon behaviour, which can be confusing, somewhat bizarre or aggressive and frightening. There are now some serious questions being asked to explore whether these challenging forms of behaviour might be attempts at some form of self-expression or communication. There is a discernable shift in the approach of some carers which is now concerned more with under-standing and interpreting behaviour rather than with management and control, but as one person noted 'it is often easy to understand why a patient is wandering or shouting, but it is not always easy to deal with it'. This chapter is concerned with that issue.

A consultant psychiatrist wrote in suggesting that when people are not heard they may become irritable or even aggressive, and he quoted the words of Martin Luther King, 'violence is the voice of the unheard'. This may account, he said, for why people with dementia are aggressive in some settings but not in others. I was interested to explore to what extent challenging behaviour was seen as a form of communication. A colleague reading through some of my material confessed to being misled at the start by the term 'challenging behaviour'. He assumed that it was describing a technique by which carers challenged the behaviour of people with dementia. The challenge, of course, is to us who are being challenged to interpret the behaviour, cope with it or live with it. My consultative document put it this way:

> We know that people's behaviour, whatever form it takes, is very often an attempt to express something which they are unable to articulate verbally. For instance, wandering or shouting may not simply be a function of the illness. People with dementia may be trying to express

their feelings by behaviour patterns which we find difficult to understand or cope with.

Difficult or challenging behaviour is a rather neglected area of study and reflection, a point brought out by Teri *et al.* (1992)

> Behaviour disturbance is a critical and understudied aspect of Alzheimer's disease. Alzheimer's disease is not just a disease of the memory. It is a disease characterised by significant and devastating behavioural impairments. Their association with other aspects of the disease process, their potential importance in etiology and progression, and their clinical management is desperately needed. (p.86)

There are many factors that make people behave in the way that they do and, at different times and in different places, one or more of these will be more predominant than others. In the case of people with dementia it is extremely important that we understand this and that we are able to tease out the varying factors and recognise their influence at any one particular time. Our behaviour is a result of the combination of our personality, our experiences of the past (sometimes specifically and sometimes collectively), the way in which we are being treated at the moment, our physical context and environment, our general health and sense of well-being and, in the case of people with dementia, the specific neurological impairments that our particular illness brings.

One of the distressing aspects of dementia is that for so many people, but not for all, it prompts behaviour which can range from the bizarre to the frightening. This is often called difficult or problematic behaviour, but increasingly is being described as *challenging behaviour* because it presents a real challenge to us to know how best to understand it and react to it. When the person is living at home, the behaviour of the person with dementia can mean that carers have disturbed days and nights and they often feel extremely stressed and distressed. There may be occasions of social embarrassment and over time the strains that such behaviour cause can led to a deterioration or to a decisive change in their patterns of relationships. This process is often called, and it can sometimes be a very apt term, a 'living bereavement' – but it is not always so.

When a person is brought into care, or is receiving domiciliary services, their behaviour can at times have quite an effect upon those who are providing the service. They will invariably suffer some form of frustration and may feel helpless, anxious or 'a failure' in their inability to cope as effectively and as creatively as they would wish. There may be a concern for other people, which means that the carer has to weigh the demands of one against the demands of the other. What often happens, though not always, is that workers develop negative feelings towards people whose behaviour is consistently perceived to be antisocial, and they may resort to ignoring them, leading them away from where things are happening and leaving them. Alternatively, they may use various forms of constraints including drugs. But the scenario is not always negative, and there are occasions and places where people adapt to these forms of behaviour with creativity and immense tenderness and goodwill. McGregor and Bell (1994) enthuse about the challenge:

> So long as the living environment is designed so that our residents are safe, then on a day to day basis they can be given the opportunity to make their own decisions about what they want to do, and how they are going to live their lives. It is a source of great pleasure and fun that the people with dementia we care for are so unpredictable and individual…this may, of course, prove overwhelmingly difficult for the carer struggling on their own, but for a specialist unit, the result is a whole community which is buzzing and dynamic. (p.20)

It is fairly common practice to apply the ABC technique to challenging behaviour. First take a close look at the *activating* event, or the *antecedent* to the behaviour. What seemed to bring it about? Then look at the actual *behaviour* itself, and then consider the *consequences* of the behaviour. But the important question, from our point of view, is to ask: *Is the person trying to communicate something to us by this behaviour?* Is the behaviour itself a form of communication? From the replies that came in, there certainly seems to be a gut feeling with many people that perhaps there might be more to the behaviour than at first meets the eye. However, there are still approaches which seem more concerned with controlling and settling the person down rather than understanding what lies behind the behaviour, as this comment from a medical practitioner shows:

> challenging behaviour can be extremely disrupting and ward nurses often react by distancing themselves and isolating the patient as a short-term manoeuvre. This often works and saves prescribing psychotropic medication. Certainly removal of the patient into a quieter environment with much less visual and auditory stimulation can be of value in quietening a patient who has moved from vocally challenging behaviour towards physical aggression, and it is one means of dealing with the situation in general wards.

Of course, the first and immediate task is to deal with the situation as it presents itself, but the above comment fails to suggest that there is a next step, which is to ascertain just why the person behaved in this way. However, as a charge nurse commented, 'it is often easy to understand why a patient is wandering or shouting, but it is not always easy to deal with it'.

The deputy manager of a home for older people felt that there was a challenge to care in this sort of behaviour and was prepared to take up that challenge:

> I am increasingly feeling that any behaviour that we either don't understand or find difficult must be interpreted. I spend a lot of time with staff saying 'what else might this mean?', when their literal response fails.

> One lady repeated the words 'help me' over and over again. When the question was answered literally with comments like 'what would you like me to do?', or 'what do you need?' the client was unable to identify anything. After numerous responses like this the staff gave up responding, but the 'help me's' continued. When we explored this we realised that the words had a much deeper meaning, along the lines of 'help me to find myself again'. We then bypassed the question and simply gave attention even if it was just a smile and a wave every time she asked for help. We agreed not to ask her to identify what she wanted, as she seemed unable to identify anything and this often led to a feeling of friction and was quite oppressive. It also gave the staff the fuel they needed to write the behaviour off as 'attention seeking'. This approach went a long way to reducing the behaviour and on many occasions the 'help me's' were followed by a specific request.

> There is no doubt in my mind that these alternative responses can only come through discussion with people doing the caring. They are not literal or obvious responses and we only reach them through thinking beyond the problem and interpreting behaviour.

An unusual point was made by a retired clinical psychologist who wrote:

> My experience with other client groups tells me that 'bad' behaviour is likely to be an expression of fear, anger or frustration, or is a valid response to the way that the world is perceived by the individual. The notion of the behaviour being a valid response to the phenomenal world of the individual seems particularly interesting as it seems likely that he is 'misperceiving' (by our criteria!) his environment. Do we know much yet about the generalities (if any) or individual concepts/perceptions of their immediate world?

As one other person commented, quoting Professor Bernard Isaacs, people with dementia are trying to behave logically – the challenge is to tap into that logic!

Exploring this whole issue made obvious sense to the sister/manager of a day care centre, who made this contribution:

> I applaud your term 'challenging behaviour', so often described as 'aggressive behaviour'. I often refer to it as 'frustration'. We must understand that people losing their ability to verbally express themselves frequently experience people talking *for* and *about* them. They are often treated as if they have no emotions and are not supposed to feel angry or bad-tempered because they have dementia. We all 'get out of bed on the wrong side' some days. A process of elimination can rule out physical discomfort, for instance headache, constipation, urinary tract infections or sore feet. Other factors like the environment need to be examined, and what happened prior to the 'behaviour'. Is the person experiencing hallucinations? Another cause may be embarrassment.

> One lady attender has an awareness that her speech is defective and in particular has word-finding difficulties. Reality Orientation groups are particularly threatening to her and she can become very irritated when asked questions. We have learned not to include her in such activities but found that she enjoys quizzes when questions are directed to a group. Another lady became frustrated when playing bingo because her numeracy skills were declining.

> People with dementia still have their pride and it is important to provide activities which do not make them feel demoralised. Whenever a member becomes angry, irritated or starts to shout we always attempt to take them into a quiet area to reduce their embarrassment and reduce any stress to the other members.

Challenging behaviour rarely occurs without a reason, commented a patient services manager, and 'undesirable behaviour should always be examined in context. It is very important to *understand* behaviour, and here, when time allows, we attempt a behavioural analysis'. A staff nurse added a common-sense note when she remarked: 'with any problem behaviour, if it doesn't pose a direct threat, it isn't a problem'.

Once again there were many requests for further training. There is need for it, if the secretary of a local Alzheimer's Disease Society branch is right:

Challenging behaviour from someone with dementia is often a sign of frustration in that people are not listening to them and, in the case of service providers, totally ignoring them.

One of the problems highlighted by a customer services manager was that

dementia has a low status with professionals. More skilled and able professionals are required who can interpret the challenging behaviour and offer advice to carers and relatives. It is essential that the right interpretation of behaviour takes place. It may be an expression of frustration. Because people are unable to interpret the behaviour and respond accordingly, the behaviour may continue to deteriorate.

Wandering

Wandering behaviour is very common amongst people with dementia; perhaps between a third and a half of all people diagnosed are reported to display this kind of behaviour at some time or other, and it can be extremely distressing for relatives and for all who care for them. Kate Allan (1994) wrote that:

it is one of the most challenging behavioural problems in dementia, making demands upon the coping skills even of those with extensive training and experience in the field. When people who wander have to be cared for in settings which are not geared to dealing with the behaviour and the problems it can cause, the resulting strain and anxiety can be enormous…wandering is a complex and challenging behaviour demanding an individualised and imaginative approach. Although there are no straightforward solutions, careful observation and thoughtful interventions can reduce wandering, or remove the need for it. (pp.32, 34)

There are various questions which can be asked immediately in order to bring some structure to thinking about this form of behaviour. Does the wandering take place alone, or in the company of others? Is it apparently aimless or are there clear objectives? Is it just the walking which is a problem or does it include other problems as well – such as being inappropriately dressed? What is the emotional state of the person as they wander? Is wandering a continuous problem or does it tend to be episodic?

A senior social worker expressed the view that

> wandering is very difficult to cope with because it is difficult to stop and has no respect for the personal space of others;

whilst a professor in the care of the elderly expressed the conviction that

> challenging behaviour always has an underlying cause and often this relates to a failure of normal communication. It is not adequate, for example, just to consider a person as a wanderer. There are very many different patterns of wandering and careful observation will often shed considerable insight into the cause of a behavioural change.

Research done by Hussian in 1982 provided evidence to suggest that wandering was not a random activity. In mapping the routes of three wanderers over a period of time in a residential setting, he found that 59 per cent of stops were within one foot of another person or of a group of people, and that 29 per cent of stops were at windows that had an external view and that 5 per cent were at isolated chairs. Thus, 93 per cent of all wandering journeys made by these three 'known wanderers' seemed to lead to a logical destination. The question for us to ask is – is this predilection for wandering behaviour actually trying to tell us something? Is it an attempt to convey something which words can no longer convey? To talk about 'aimless wandering' involves a judgment on our part that the person concerned does not have a definite purpose to their walking. McGregor and Bell (1994) argue:

> Genuine 'aimless' wandering only occurs when people are sedated. People with dementia rarely set off without a purpose, they are always anxious to go somewhere specific, for their own good reasons. For instance, they may believe that they must get home to prepare tea for their children returning from school, or that they need to look after their parents who are ill... (p.21)

What carers need is the capacity to be able to cope with the behaviour, and then the skill to be able to interpret the reason behind it, and the ability to respond in such a way as to reassure the person and calm their anxieties – not by distracting them but by resolving what inner conflict sparked off the behaviour in the first place.

Aggression

Holden (1994) says that:

> Aggression is very hard to tolerate and can cause staff to feel afraid or deeply insulted. Invariably the situation results in feelings of dislike toward the patient – or at least extreme caution. It is very difficult to know how to manage such behaviour and how best to provide the necessary care. (p.37)

She goes on to say that 'there is always an explanation for aggressive outbursts or verbal abuse'; the challenge is, of course, to discover what that explanation is, and to see what it might be attempting to communicate to us. She suggests possible explanations for aggression, which might arise from confusion over a number of different factors, such as:

- Misunderstanding personal care as an intrusion into personal privacy.
- The person having some insight into their condition and trying to cope with it and hide it from others.
- Being unable to perform a particular task and becoming increasingly frustrated by the process.
- Not being able to come to terms with an environment which may appear to be strange and may be perceived as threatening.
- Poor eyesight, poor hearing or interrupted sleep patterns may make a person prone to misunderstandings.
- Staffing may be perceived (and experienced) as being aggressive or threatening and provoke a defensive reaction.
- The person may be expected to do or receive things which they perceive as being inappropriate.

Or there may be specific precipitating factors, such as:

- There is not sufficient stimulation or conversation in the environment.
- The physical environment may be unhelpful in terms of there not being clear directional signs, or there being insufficient information, or the rooms being too hot or too cold, or having limited privacy, etc.
- Feeling that remaining skills are being overlooked, and therefore feeling a pressure to become even more dependent.
- Complaints being ignored or decisions being made with insufficient consultation or explanation.

- ◦ A lack of consistency in personal care, with too many different people being involved.
- ◦ Different carers having different approaches.
- ◦ Noise and disturbances disrupting sleep patterns.
- ◦ Specific happenings which cause the person to feel a loss of status or which fail to address them as a unique individual.
- ◦ Physical restraint or inappropriate medication.

A project manager wrote in saying:

> I am always amazed that there is not a lot more aggression in dementia care environments. I think the fear, frustration and panic of living and drowning in a wave of cognitive disruption must surely lead to the aggression of desperation. For example, I remember a client who could no longer speak, but at that time could still walk. She had two 'words' in her emotional vocabulary; to hit or to hug. I learned this the hard way when she hit me so hard that she almost broke my arm. Afterwards I initiated hugs, as this gave us both pleasure – and was safer! She became even more distressed if she had hit someone, because I am sure she did not want to add to the sum total of suffering.
>
> It is very hard to do, but I think we have to recognise people's right to anger, that in their position it is often an appropriate response, and therefore healthy.

Another contributor from a residential home commented that

> challenging behaviour is often interpreted by staff as aggressive behaviour. It is frightening. Encouraging staff to give alternative explanations for this behaviour allows them to see what is really happening – what the person is trying to communicate to us. If challenging behaviour is handled wrongly, then client frenzy may develop – I see this as an example of carer failure. Not all challenging behaviour is psychological in origin – there may be physical problems – pain, needing to go to the toilet and unable to find it, being wet and uncomfortable, constipation etc.... If challenging behaviour is psychological in origin, this may be due to an inability to locate the self in time and place. It is based on fear and anxiety. Calm acceptance and reassurance is effective. I suppose that the best way of dealing with extremes of this type of behaviour is not to let it develop! This is not to say that residents should not have quarrels, voice their views loudly etc. – it is the frenzied and aggressive behaviours which are upsetting for everyone.

A clinical nurse specialist, dealing with early onset dementia wrote:

> I have a gentleman I visit who is unable to communicate verbally. By
> using nonverbal techniques I feel he is able to communicate with me
> and vice versa. He likes to pat people on the shoulder etc., and this is
> often received as threatening to those with little understanding. It is
> my experience that this is his way of making contact and saying 'hello'.
> It was initially deemed challenging behaviour but is now seen as it
> really is – an attempt to communicate.

A senior nurse for mental health made the point that

> if instead of looking at behaviour exhibited by people with dementia
> as problems we look at them as messages, we will gain much more. If
> we look at aggression as a message that either the person has not
> understood what is happening or does not like what is happening, we
> are more likely to resolve it rather than if we just label the person
> 'aggressive'.

Another person commented that he knew a man who became abusive and
aggressive when he was forced to wear incontinence pads. When they were
left off he became calm and contented. This respondent also quoted a lady
who would sing a nonsense rhyme over and over again in a most raucous
voice. One day she said, quite lucidly, 'Why don't you stop me doing it? It's
more interesting when you stop me!'

The importance of knowing life histories

Several people commented how they were perplexed about certain types of
behaviour until they remembered or discovered key facts about the person's
earlier life, then suddenly the behaviour patterns became much more understandable and manageable. A services manager wrote:

> concentrating on one client's life story – of intense activity as a crofter,
> allowed staff to recognise that his early morning agitation was a result
> of inactivity. A programme of accompanied morning walks followed
> by gradual integration into organised activity groups eased the
> difficulties.

A project co-ordinator shared this example:

> We had a resident who fought, bit and scratched and kicked staff who
> tried to take her to the toilet. Toileting needed to be done as the lady
> had lost the ability to look after herself. The staff found this a difficult

and degrading exercise until we were informed that our resident had been raped as a young woman. Although this information did not change the resident's behaviour it did have an effect on the staff who could now understand her difficult behaviour, and respect her for this.

Another project co-ordinator explained how knowing about a person's background made it easier for them to cope. She wrote:

> we helped one lady who to onlookers with no understanding of dementia appeared to be an aggressive, malicious old lady. However, we helped her for two years with no problems because we understood her fear and frustration etc., and her life history which told us that she used to be a gentle, loving woman.

Developing coping strategies

Many of the people who wrote in described how they approached dealing with challenging behaviour, and how they persisted in struggling in order that they might eventually find some hidden clue as to why the person behaved in the way that they did. Once some form of order is restored there is the even greater challenge of trying to discover just why the person was behaving in that way, and trying to understand what the behaviour might mean. I was interested in reading about different people's coping strategies. A senior physiotherapist wrote:

> we need to look beyond the outward behaviours that people display. I work in a day hospital for older people with mental health difficulties. We are often having to deal with clients who are angry, sometimes verbally aggressive and agitated. As a team we have learned to handle these situations. Things are often worse at the end of the day as transport is due to take the clients home. The majority of their actions are due to anxiety about getting home again or worried about what time they will return or fearful that their relatives may not know where they are. Understanding this helps us to remain patient, reassuring and calm. There is no alternative but to know each individual well and what in particular makes them anxious. Also, everyone in the team takes responsibility for assisting if we see someone getting anxious or agitated (from consultant to receptionist) and this helps to ease the strain from the day hospital staff.

A principal officer for the elderly and physically disabled wrote in saying that there are many ways in which people with dementia do try to express themselves and challenging behaviour is certainly one of them. It is enormously frustrating for people who feel their relative, carer, worker, does not understand what they are trying to say. It is certainly not well enough understood that aggression, crying, distress and antisocial behaviour may all be part of the pattern of people with dementia trying to express their emotions and thoughts. Unfortunately in some residential care the way that difficult and challenging behaviour is dealt with is by the 'liquid cosh'. This in some cases is an easy way to deal with this behaviour rather than by trying to understand it.

An inspector recognised that even understanding what causes challenging behaviour may not be enough to resolve it and cause the person to behave in a more socially acceptable manner. For some people, it was better to separate them out into specialist units:

> whilst recognising that separate residential units for people with challenging behaviour might be seen as stigmatising, most people were clear that it gave a positive experience to residents in those units. What was helpful perhaps was the opportunity to concentrate training on a small dedicated staff group who were then more able to concentrate on the special needs of their residents.

> One other point that has been made to me over and over again, comes from the carers' group who point out that they often have the experience of managing people with challenging behaviour, borne out of their long experience of that person. Too often, they say, we the professionals ignore this expertise.

A development officer wrote:

> in our centre 'challenging behaviour' was always seen as a form of communication and staff would always try to interpret this, attempting to tune into a person's feeling or distress. People who 'wandered' were never told to sit down, but staff time was spent with them. A useful resource here is an enclosed garden or conservatory. ABC analysis may assist in helping to recognise triggers. Staff may build up a 'bank' of appropriate responses based on experience. Important you don't try to suppress the behaviour (in Dementia Care Mapping terms this would be seen as a negative response), but manage the distress.

A director of clinical development commented that

> when things go wrong in our lives we all feel like screaming and shouting. Giving the person space to scream, being non-judgmental

about such behaviour and providing reassurance that they are still a valued person is a form of 'listening' to the sufferer's message.

The manager of a day care centre outlined her approach:

> challenging behaviour is often the result of frustration in unsuccessful attempts at communication. We should attempt to interpret this form of communication and not dismiss it out of hand as aggression or awkward behaviour. Sometimes the only way to understand this form of communication is to re-enact the situations until each variable has been analysed and eliminated and the root cause isolated.

The search for the elusive clue which can open up the situation was emphasised by an advisor to a team for services for older people, who wrote:

> I usually find touch (e.g. on the forearm) useful to reassure people or gain their attention. I have seen music have an amazing effect. For example, one lady I tested who had been non-communicative (no facial expression, just a 'depressed' posture) for years, suddenly leaped to her feet and sang 'Men of Harlech' all through in Welsh when the music was played! It's all about finding the right trigger for enabling communication to take place.

A development nurse in dementia services responded to this part of the consultative document by saying:

> this factor cannot be emphasised enough. I spend a large amount of time discussing this with ward staff who have asked to have teaching on *management* of aggression, or *management* of repetitive speech, or *control* of someone who is wandering. The hardest aspect to put across is that we should stop trying to manage, control or continue to have a power relationship over the person and start really looking at that behaviour more closely. Not just looking, but really 'seeing' and making the connections tangible. I have found that giving specific case studies detailing the challenging behaviour and explaining the reasons for *that* individual, often puts things into context for the professional carers who will then be more likely to take it on board. I also emphasise that this sort of thing is always a learning experience because individuals do differ, so sometimes we will make mistakes. If we live and learn from our mistakes then they will become more infrequent and the carer who is really 'looking' will find communicating with a person with dementia a satisfying and enriching experience.

Starting with ourselves

What was very obvious, in reading through the many submissions on this subject, was that very often *we* have a problem in coming to terms with challenging behaviour, and perhaps our first task is to acknowledge what we ourselves are thinking and experiencing. Only then will we be sufficiently free to be able to give the person with dementia our full attention. As one carer put it:

> what we all need to do is to cope with and recognise the shortcomings of our own reactions to challenging behaviour. Once we can accept and understand it without being embarrassed, we will take great steps forward in communicating with people with dementia.

A human resource development manager put it this way:

> working with staff about problems caused to them by such challenging behaviours as inappropriate sexuality [see e.g. Archibald 1994] and verbal and physical violence it is clear that they need to understand the client's history and their own self awareness needs to be increased. They need to know what may trigger the violence or other behaviour in the client and what feelings it may evoke in themselves, and ideally, why they have these reactions themselves.

Which brings me to the final point which came up time and time again, and that was for more training and help in knowing how to respond more creatively to challenging behaviour, so that staff are better able to accept it as a possible attempt to communicate and may have the skills and the confidence to respond appropriately.

CHAPTER 12

Group Work

> To what extent can communication be encouraged and facilitated by skilled group work? It would appear that this is a question which is hardly being addressed in Britain at the moment. There is evidence from Scandinavia and from the United States to suggest that this is a very creative and positive area to explore. It is, however, costly in terms of time and staff resources. Group work in Britain tends to be limited to interest and/or recreational ends at the moment, but a small yet significant number of people are now wanting to do more intensive therapeutic work with people with dementia – at all stages of their illness.

Even when communication seems very difficult, it is sometimes possible to encourage and stimulate people with dementia in such a way as to facilitate conversation and discover their views and preferences. Sometimes in such a process restless behaviour is reduced and a sense of well-being seems to increase. Some imaginative work has been done with people with dementia in small groups, and ways have been found of encouraging people to set their own agendas in such groups.

A literature search had revealed some interesting work being done in Scandinavia and in the United States and I was interested to discover if much work was being done in this field in Britain. My consultative document therefore asked people if they had experience of working with people in small groups in ways which enabled them to develop their own themes and express their feelings. I was also interested to learn if much work was being done with people in later stages of their illness.

There were considerably fewer responses to this set of questions, and the overall impression that they gave was that most people were in the very early stages of thinking about using group work in any systematic, developmental way. There were numerous examples of people enjoying a singsong, but not many explorations of the process that was taking place when people gathered together for some sort of activity. Nor were there many suggestions that much therapeutic work was being embarked upon, although there were some indications that here and there this was being explored.

A Scandinavian experience

My interest in the subject was stimulated by reading an article by Britt Mari Akerlund and Astrid Norberg (1986). Working in Sweden, they reflected on the fact that elderly people with dementia have traditionally been regarded as being beyond the reach of psychotherapeutic methods, but noted that attempts were being made to find alternative ways of treating them. Life review, reality orientation and reminiscence therapy were increasingly being used but, according to Akerlund and Norberg, evaluation of these approaches has been somewhat ambiguous. They felt therefore a strong need to find new methods 'to improve or at least maintain' the person's fading cognitive and emotional functions. They embarked upon a study in 1983 in which they changed a reality orientation group into a psychodynamically oriented group, after asking themselves two basic questions:

- Is it possible to improve the cognitive functions of people in an advanced state of dementia through reality orientation?
- Are there methods to stimulate their remaining mental functions that do not focus on their deteriorating memory?

This second question was raised because the patients seemed to be discouraged when they realised that memory was continuing to fail.

The patients were encouraged to introduce their own topics for discussion, and the groups were led by a psychiatric nurse and a psychologist working as co-therapists who restricted their participation to supporting dialogue between group members. 'Eventually the therapists interpreted for them the emotional content in their conversations' (p.83). What they discovered was that the patients became more actively involved and their conversation was on a higher cognitive and emotional level than in the earlier reality orientation groups. 'The patients' feelings of anxiety, forsakenness, anger, longing, despair and hope became the topics of conversation. A woman who was the wanderer sat still through the ninety minute session' (p.84). It became obvious to the group leaders that the group had changed, and so they then brought in a third person to analyse what was happening from videotapes which they made of the group sessions.

The small pilot group consisted of three patients who were severely demented and one who was much more severely demented. Five hour-long sessions were videotaped and the sessions analysed. In the first session the group members told each other about how much they missed their spouses, and how lonely life was for them at the hospital. Another session focused on faithfulness and they spoke of their fears that their partners may not be being faithful to them whilst they were in hospital. A further session revolved around their feelings about their own illness and their fear of death – 'their descriptions of their own experiences during illness demonstrated insight into their situation. The atmosphere was appropriately sombre' (p.84).

Summing up the study Akerlund and Norberg (1986) comment that

> the most striking difference between the reality orientation group and the psychodynamic pilot group was the amount of verbal activity by severely demented patients. [They] interacted with each other and responded to each other more frequently. In the reality orientation group patients responded only to questions from the group leader…how and why a dynamic approach can improve demented patients' behaviour are questions that require more thorough analysis. However, this small pilot study on the psychodynamic approach has at least cast more light on our understanding of severely demented patients and given us a possible means to discover their concealed memories, thoughts and feelings. (p.84)

British experience

Given this interesting start, I wondered what experiences people had of such groups in Britain. Most of the respondents outlined more general group work, such as these examples:

- People with dementia have been involved in attending art therapy groups successfully. We include them in group discussions within the residential setting but are unable, at present, to estimate the value of the exercise. (*services manager*)
- My contact with a community mental health team for older people revealed that one of the most successful groups run by the team was a group for men with dementia living with spouses in the community. This was structured around a mixture of an occupational therapist workshop, a cup of tea and lunch, and a 'group session' when a lot of work was done of a highly 'therapeutic' and/or personal expressive nature, with the men voicing (apparently very eloquently from reports of the group leaders) concerns about

sexuality, death, the relationship with their spouse and the loss of functioning and its impact on them. (*researcher*)

○ Residents are individually assessed and then work in groups of approximately six or seven, of the same or similar ability levels, with one staff member to aid interaction. Activities are set for the group's ability level to encourage success and a feeling of self-worth – they are not set out to make anyone feel a failure. Groups are smaller, three or four people, for people in latter stages of dementia. Cluster groups encourage participation and interaction, enabling a higher quality of life and maintaining individual skills. (*manager*)

○ There is a tendency to hear only the voice of the carer. We have a Memory Therapy Group run by occupational therapists that enables clients to express their feelings and share ways of coping. There have also been groups for people in early dementia that are single sex, which is seen as enabling. (*senior mental health practitioner*)

○ I carried out a survey of a group of five day care patients who were transported by the non-Emergency Ambulance Service, using Critical Incident Technique, which was very successful. At first one lady dominated the conversation but she gradually drew the others in by asking them direct questions herself, and by the end the whole group were joining in the discussion and giving examples of how caring the staff were and also how upsetting it was to be collected early from the Centre. In fact it was this experience which convinced me of the power of the CIT technique in improving quality. (*research and development specialist – quality*)

○ We have various group work activities which we feel are beneficial for our residents with dementia, apart from our residents meetings. Music, cooking, exercise classes. Water therapy we have found to be very beneficial in the late stages of dementia. We have two or three forms of this at present – Jacuzzi, foot spa and playing with various objects in the water. (*director of nursing services*)

○ Success depends upon the skills and expertise of group leaders and support that they have from other carers in convening the group. I have indirect experience of a small group for men with moderate dementia. They assembled late morning for a woodwork session with a male occupational therapist technician followed by lunch and an hour-long group facilitated by an experienced community psychiatric nurse and occupational therapist. The group was eventually able to focus on issues including the change of status and role that the group members had experienced within their own families and on their anxieties about their cognitive losses and the sense that they were nearing the end of their life span. It was felt that none of the group members could have engaged in this sort of discussion on an individual basis. (*clinical psychology section head*)

○ In a previous post I used group work to stimulate awareness of others and to assist creative expression. A favourite of group members was to compose a free-style verse by selecting a subject and using pictures or objects as an aid to help the group each say something about what that meant to them. By recording such statements some very powerful poems which expressed the people's feelings were produced. (*staff nurse*)

North American experience

Much work in this field is currently being done in the United States by Robyn Yale (1993a). She writes that the classically recognised 'curative factors' of group therapy are all relevant to people with Alzheimer's disease, including:

○ *the instillation of hope* – life can still have meaning and quality despite the diagnosis

○ *universality* – a person does not have to be alone in facing this disease

○ *imparting of information* – concerning both resources which are available and also biomedical knowledge

○ *altruism* – there can still be a concern for others, which can be expressed

○ *socialisation* – it is possible to meet and mix with others – deficits can be tolerated

○ *cohesiveness* – people are brought together and can identify with one another when they struggle with similar symptoms

○ *interpersonal learning* – sharing coping strategies with each other

○ *existential factors* – learning how to face up to one's own mortality.

She refers to work done in recent years with terminally ill people who have cancer and how many of them are brought to a point where they can begin to grieve in a healthy way, as they come to terms with their diagnosis and the inevitability of death. We do not yet know whether people with Alzheimer's disease are able to accomplish this and so, she says, 'because the level of insight and intellectual capacity are difficult to ascertain, professionals may inaccurately assume that patients are *not* capable of an individualised grief reaction' (p.9). However, Yale believes that many people with Alzheimer's disease do communicate to their carers, in many different ways, what they want to know and can assimilate, and that they make their limits known to them. Her work proceeds on the basis that

> patients who learn about the Alzheimer's diagnosis with peers in a similar situation may then be better equipped to face the crisis together with their family members. Those who ask for information are likely to grieve and cope in more maladaptive ways if they are denied the opportunity for open discussion (p.10).

She therefore runs a number of groups for people with dementia where they are able to discuss their diagnosis and their hopes and fears for the future.

If a person understands their diagnosis, then there is a chance that their autonomy can be maximised by their participation in decision-making. Yale says that this allows for at least some sense of control over what can otherwise feel like 'helpless victimisation by the disease'. It is the relationship amongst the participants of a group which becomes the major therapeutic tool, and

> despite disruptions due to forgetfulness, group members overall displayed patience, curiosity, empathy, and a remarkable ability to articulate their feelings and experiences...over time they became more comfortable sharing such feelings as humiliation due to the need for supervision, helplessness, sadness and worry...patients talked about the things they were no longer able to do, and how they compensated for them...ultimately they shared their recognition that they needed to make fewer demands upon and be more patient and loving with themselves (p.42).

Elsewhere (Yale 1993b) she has listed the sort of subjects which came up in these groups. These include feelings of stigma, changes in lifestyle and responsibilities, issues relating to driving a car, dependency, issues with their families (they often felt that their families did not understand that certain behaviours were due to their illness – as one said, 'I don't do these things on purpose'), relationships with friends, problems of communication, their attitudes towards research into the illness, their sense of well-being and optimism and preparing for the future.

In general

In the light of all these instances, it is interesting to reflect that several people wrote to me saying that group work does not work. 'I feel that group work confronts the dementia sufferer with their own shortcomings, causing distress and sometimes anger,' said one ward manager, whilst a head occupational therapist said that it might work in the early stages but 'it doesn't work with clients in middle to later stages of dementia. They seem to perceive only themselves amongst strangers'.

However, a senior nurse for mental health commented that 'nobody is too badly damaged mentally not to enjoy group work'. A sister in an elderly mentally infirm unit enthused about group work saying that 'communication greatly increased, even for a person suffering from the later stage of dementia', and a clinical services manager reported that 'we have found one of the most successful types of group work is in-depth reminiscence work. This usually stimulates conversation within the group'. An officer in charge of a home seemed to be well on the way to being convinced about group work, but just needed a little more encouragement – she wrote:

> I feel that group work with clients suffering the full effects of dementia needs more investigation. Often I feel we do little more than 'maintain' a person. Often, just by matching people with things in common who have similar disabilities can help people converse or at times just 'wander' together. At best a meaningful conversation can ensue; at worst people can find physical comfort by sitting close to someone.

A clinical psychologist recognised the value of group work, but pointed out that it is very labour intensive when working with people who have severe dementia; even so it was interesting to note that quite a number of people were thinking in terms of introducing or extending group work. A development nurse in dementia services wrote:

> this is a subject which really interests me. Currently we have no group work facilities, but this is another of my objectives for [the current year]. I would like to have small group work running on a regular basis and believe that this is achievable in spite of the ward workload and the severity of the dementing process in our patients. I am looking at how I can utilise the best ideas from Reminiscence/Validation therapy and Reality Orientation in a manner that best suits each individual, and feel that purposeful interactions like these will reduce the staff workload because patients are less likely to resort to challenging behaviour in order to communicate. Staff members who contribute will learn an immeasurable amount about the individual patients and further develop their own communication strategies. The knock-on effect should improve patients' feelings of well-being throughout the hospital admission and not just during the group work, as well as contribute even further to the accuracy and efficacy of the life histories (and vice versa).

There is something really pleasurable in sensing someone's excitement at the prospect of developing this sort of work, who can see the long-term possibilities far outweighing the immediate problems of workload and the deteriorating condition of the people with whom she works. A further positive response came from a consultant clinical psychologist, who said, 'in our service, some small group work does take place, with benefit to those participating. We are anxious to try to extend this to people with dementia whose command of language is more limited'.

A resource worker with the Alzheimer's Society was keen to develop this type of work, writing:

> I have seen group work being used very effectively for people with dementia. It tends to be more effective in smaller groups and with skilled people leading the group. As people are being diagnosed at an earlier age and are being told the diagnosis, this is an issue which needs to be discussed more widely. The possibility of bringing people together with similar problems is one which is very real for people with other illnesses and we certainly need to be looking at that for people with dementia.

A clinical psychologist wrote in saying that he did not have any experience of small group work with people with dementia but he did have experience of this kind of work with people with severe learning disabilities, and from that experience he offered the following advice:

- The group must be very small
- The group worker often has to repeat any communication clearly and directly to another group member, and prompt a response. This, in turn, then has to be repeated back to the first speaker
- Initially, even a simple response is an achievement
- Stick to simple, short communications
- Tie the communication to practical situations of known common interest, and use objects, visual and auditory aids
- Be incredibly patient and not discouraged early or easily.

Now all groups are different and all this advice may not be relevant to each and every group, but the important thing is that he encourages us to stick at it and not be put off when things may, at first, seem very difficult. Once again there are training implications. Staff need to develop the skills to be able to observe, hear what is being said *and* what is not being said, and also to have confidence and patience. Group work of this nature is not the same as drawing a few people together for an afternoon chat – although that too is often a beneficial activity. This sort of group work believes that it is possible for people to communicate, and it recognises that sometimes it requires considerable skill to enable people to do this and for their communications to be received and honoured.

Testing out an hypothesis

Gordon Lockerbie of Grampian Social Work Department in Scotland under-took a project specifically to answer the question 'Does a programme of group work in a specialist setting improve specific behaviours in people with dementia?'.[1] The project lasted three months, and amongst the findings he reported that:

- Some specific behaviours were consistently more relaxed and less agitated during groups when directly compared to out of group behaviour.
- During groups, significant improvements in behaviour were related to reductions in wandering, repeated questioning and requests to go home, as well as improvements in orientation for time and place and increased socialisation.
- Similar improvements between 4pm and 8pm were noted for wandering, questioning and requests to go home, but not in orientation and socialisation. (This was the time when staff had reported challenging behaviour incidents increased).
- Following the end of the project and a subsequent period of non-group activity, deterioration in cognitive functioning was recorded.

He concluded that

> the results indicate the benefits of group work for people with dementia. The consequence for staff is that they can spend their time working constructively and imaginatively in the best interests of their clients, as opposed to frequently responding to agitated and demanding behaviour which occurs when clients are not involved in group activities. The benefits for the person with dementia...suggest the value of group work becoming accepted practice in other residential settings with a dementia population.

---

1   Further details from Gordon Lockerbie, Birse Unit, Social Work Department, Allachburn, Aboyne AB34 5HF.

Conclusion

I have a growing conviction that this is going to be an important area of growth in the next decade. Given the suspicion about psychotherapy and therapeutic group work in society at large it is perhaps not surprising that not a great deal of work has been undertaken with people with dementia. As people become more aware of the subjective experience of dementia then there are bound to be issues to be resolved and anxieties and fears to be worked through. So long as people with dementia were considered to be unaware of their situation, there seemed to be little need to explore these subjects. That scenario is changing. I believe that therapeutic group work will soon become an important, if not essential, element in good dementia care.

CHAPTER 13

To Tell or Not to Tell –
is That the Question?

> *More differences of opinion were expressed on issues relating to sharing a diagnosis of dementia than on any other part of my study. The literature seems to favour an early diagnosis being given to a person, but in reality it is invariably made at a relatively late stage of the illness. Some of the arguments for and against are identified. Even if it is to be shared, there are a whole set of questions relating to how, and to when, and how often. GPs are placed in an unenviable position and some of the difficulties of making a diagnosis are looked at. And still the problems of communication remain...*

The last of the ten points raised in my consultative document brought more discussion and disagreement than any of the earlier nine. I suggested that

> if people do not know what is wrong with them, and what the development of their illness is likely to be, then how realistic is it to ask them if they are satisfied with the services being provided? Might they want different services if they knew more about their condition? In my experience very few people seem to have been told or understood their diagnosis or condition, and great collusion takes place to ensure that the word 'dementia' is not mentioned. The phrase 'problems with your memory' euphemistically covers known diagnoses. The situation with dementia seems to be where the situation with cancer was twenty years ago.

I asked people how honest we are in our dealings with people, and how we handle the thorny questions relating to colluding with the avoidance of truth? How are we able to to explore the reality of dementia with people who suffer from it with honesty and integrity if we are not allowed to discuss the illness?

An inspector wrote in reply:

> People felt that this was vital. They were particularly critical of GPs who will not share the diagnosis. This reduces our ability to work openly and honestly with both users and carers. From the carers' point of view too I know that this is one of their main pleas. Unless they are told early they cannot plan together what they want to do.

Whilst a specialist in old age psychiatry commented:

> As with all these loaded terms you need to be sure of your facts when you use them. You need to be clear whose needs you are addressing and you need to have the resources available to provide the back-up if sharing a difficult diagnosis in full seems to be what is required. To some extent you can make it possible for people to ask and know *as much as they wish to ask and know*. What is the truth anyway? A group of disorders that we are a long way from understanding, that we often diagnose by exclusion, whose manifestations and time course we can't always manage let alone predict. One of the most troublesome aspects is that the disorder undermines those skills that you need in order to cope with such a major life event. Sometimes the only certainty there is, is that knowing you have dementia is unlikely to be good news – it might be so awful that you may consider harming yourself.

Opinions amongst those who responded to the consultative document were extremely varied, but probably could be summarised by saying that carers and service providers tended to want a clear and an early diagnosis and the medical profession was much more cautious and reluctant to commit itself. However there were considerable differences of opinion within these two themselves.

Sharing the diagnosis

One of the conclusions of a literature review conducted for the Northern Ireland Dementia Policy Scrutiny (Downs *et al.* 1994) was that 'there is unanimous agreement in the literature that an early, accurate diagnosis is of benefit' (p. 1). Having said that, the report went on to say that there is actually little empirical evidence to support the claim. The view is that timely assessment is of benefit to the person with dementia because they are better able to plan for the future and also because they can have any treatable causes of impairment addressed; it is of benefit to the carer, because they are able to mobilise support and services. It is also of benefit to those people who are suffering similar symptoms, but ones which are reversible. The emphasis is on *early* diagnosis, and it seems that the later a diagnosis is made the more difficult it is to respond to it creatively in the sense that our options are rather more limited. It is also important, of course, that the diagnosis is accurate and the difficulties of making an accurate diagnosis are discussed later. So whilst the literature points to the need to share an early diagnosis the fact remains that most diagnoses are made relatively late in the course of the illness, and there is much debate about the effectiveness of sharing it at that stage.

A medical view from the United States (McGahan 1994) was that:

> While those recently diagnosed are in the process of dealing with these confusing feelings, they are still aware and mentally capable of making decisions that can affect their futures. Therefore it is important that physicians and family members respect their competency and take advantage of the positive outcomes that can be achieved, such as establishing a durable power of attorney or deciding to participate in research.

> For many people in the early stages, participating in these decisions gives them a sense of control. They have an altruistic need to make a difference, not only for themselves but for their children or future generations. (p.4)

A proprietor of a residential home summarised the situation as he found it in this way:

> We find that most people with dementia have
>
> (a) a late diagnosis, and
>
> (b) are never told what they are diagnosed as having.

> I believe that they should have the opportunity of
>
> (a) coming to terms with their illness
>
> (b) sharing it with their families and friends, and
>
> (c) preparing for their future.

A social work senior manager, who is also a carer, was quite convinced that:

> People have a right to use that knowledge to plan their future and people have the right to reject that knowledge, but it must be given to them.

A day care service manager summed up the dilemma in this way:

> I feel that people in the early stages of dementia should have their condition fully explained to them so that they have time to 'get their house in order' before the illness takes its toll. I do not see any point in telling a sufferer in the later stages what is wrong, as the memory span is so short, and the diagnosis may cause extreme distress for a short while, and so there is no reason if the sufferer is unable to act upon the information that he has received.

Even when it is recognised that there might be a different case to argue when the person with dementia is too old or whose illness is too advanced, there is still the feeling that people are not generally told their diagnosis. A principal officer for the elderly and physically disabled reflected that:

> This is something which appears to be distinctly lacking for people who are in the early stages of dementia and who can well understand what is going wrong with them. There is a hesitancy to explain to them exactly what will happen because of the fear of the reaction and also because of the need 'not to worry them'. A great deal of collusion takes place in order to ensure that the word 'dementia' is not mentioned. 'Problems with your memory' can in fact affect us all… I do not feel that the decision about telling should be left to the medical profession…unfortunately, in my experience, it is shied away from. If people know what is wrong with them, they are far more likely to express their views on the services they are going to need.

A patient services manager commented that, 'they should be told, but very rarely are in my experience. We as professionals fall down very badly in this area. It is one that we definitely need to address. Multi-disciplinary seminars might assist us to progress'. A unit manager reflected that, 'fear of the unknown is often harder to deal with than needing to come to terms with the truth and knowing what to expect of self and others'. This same point was made by a nurse whose mother has dementia, who wrote that, 'not knowing can cause more fear than knowing'; and a clinical nurse, a specialist in early onset dementia, wrote that she 'had rarely met a situation which has worsened through individuals knowing their diagnosis – in fact most of the time it improves; the uncertainty has been removed'.

Three carers had interesting perspectives on the subject:

(a) I must plead guilty to the euphemism 'problems with your memory' which my mother seemed to accept. I could not have told her that she was 'senile' which was the other phrase that she could have understood to describe her condition. On the other hand, if I was diagnosed as having dementia like my mother and grandmother, I would want to know so that all possible arrangements could be made. Times are changing!

(b) Diagnosis should be as early as possible and patients should be told of their illness immediately it is diagnosed. However, in my own experience, informing my wife was a disaster – she said repeatedly in no uncertain manner, that there was absolutely nothing wrong with her and that it was her husband, not she, who was ill!

(c) Seems rubbish. Try by all means if you have to, for your own peace of mind, but it won't help the sufferer.

The general view of the majority of respondents was that it was important that diagnoses should be shared with the person as soon as possible. The earlier the diagnosis was made the more important it was to share the information. However, it was recognised that for many people the diagnosis was made so late as to perhaps have little effect. In terms of hearing the voice of the person with dementia, and discussing with them the range and quality of services, it is obvious that the sooner a person knows the diagnosis and is able to understand and accept it, the more likely we are to be able to enter into meaningful dialogue. This is not to say that dialogue is meaningless as their condition deteriorates, but it is certainly more difficult.

Withholding the diagnosis

Whilst there is much literature to argue that diagnoses should be shared, as a matter of principle almost, there is little or no written argument for saying that people should not be told, *unless* there are specific reasons for reticence. Not sharing a diagnosis is not a matter of principle, but of expediency and judgment. It is difficult to find articles arguing for withholding information, but many of the written replies I received were rather less guarded.

> People who are suffering in the early stages of dementia are very vulnerable emotionally and being told that you have what amounts to an incurable disease may cause severe distress and anxiety. To make such a blanket statement undermines the value of a person's individual needs. (*senior manager elderly services*)

The arguments against giving an early diagnosis include:

○ A diagnosis of an illness which is irreversible and for which there is no treatment can have adverse psychological effects.

○ Dementia affects people in different ways. An early sufferer and his family will not be able to predict which behavioural changes will occur.

○ How certain is the diagnosis? A false diagnosis would seem particularly damaging.

○ People with a serious illness sometimes retain (perhaps irrationally) hope of recovery. Do professionals have the right to insist that hope is abandoned?

○ A diagnosis which in some people's eyes detracts from the individuality of the sufferer may also have bad effects on interpersonal relationships.

○ To insist that people 'face up' to their decline seems to be in the interests of the professionals rather than the sufferers. It may be a question of which of the two proverbs you prefer: 'Forewarned is forearmed,' or, 'Don't look for trouble until trouble looks for you'.

> For those families who wish for the diagnosis, both they and the patient need access to high quality supportive counselling to cope with the information and all its ramifications. Such counselling is rarely available and we suspect that there are insufficient professionals with appropriate training. Only when such support is available will it be appropriate to encourage families to give their permission for a more open approach to the truth. But, of course, there are financial implications [in providing such services]. (*Alzheimer's Society branch co-ordinator*)

A forthright view came from a senior charge nurse, who seemed to be in little doubt as to the value of withholding information about a diagnosis:

> How honest are we…how do we handle…how are we able to explore the reality of dementia? These are not the issues here. Before we indulge ourselves in navel gazing of this sort, we should be asking what is the likely effect on a person with dementia of being given this diagnosis? The implication of your statement is that people with dementia should be informed of their diagnosis in order that they may make a judgment about the services they are being offered. I find this outrageous and wholly unacceptable. These questions are secondary ones. Whose needs are we dealing with here: those of dementia sufferers, or our need to feel that we are doing a good job? Patients do not exist to satisfy our vanity or make us feel virtuous. I can imagine no clearer example of the author's concept of making the demented an 'object'.

On the one hand, patients obviously have a right to know. But even here we have a problem; given that memory impairment is a cardinal feature it is inevitable that the information will have to be imparted repeatedly. How many times are we to expect sufferers to endure this anguish?

On the other hand, it is clearly not always necessarily in the best interests of people with dementia to be given their diagnosis. To convey such potentially devastating information, particularly to someone who has not asked for it, without careful consideration of the consequences, does not constitute integrity. This decision should not be taken without the widest possible consultation, to ensure that in affording people with dementia their rights, we are not doing them a disservice.

The above quote illustrates beautifully the protectionist stance that many people develop. At best it is compassionate and sensitive, but it can also be demeaning and suggests that people are unable to handle their emotions when we know quite well that, possibly with skilled help, many people are able to do a great deal of creative work at this time of their lives, even though they may have a dementing illness. But even such a strong view as this one recognises that 'with the widest possible consultation' it might be appropriate to share a diagnosis. No one is suggesting that such a sharing should be taken lightly or handled crassly, only that it might assist in the process of dialogue if people were not protected from the truth by people acting on their behalf – and presumably without their permission to do so.

More a matter of balance

In the end it is less a matter of the importance of telling versus the importance of withholding, than it is of making a right judgment, and an appropriate response. It is a matter of balance and we are in a transition period when the emphasis is shifting from protective withholding to responsible sharing. As a consultant psychiatrist put it:

'Dementia' is a loaded word and many doctors, nurses and carers would feel that it might strike 'hopelessness' in the patient to be told this. Often the best approach is to describe in more detail – for instance, Alzheimer's disease – and outline how this might affect the individual, or describe the process such as small strokes of multi-infarct dementia. What you tell a patient will depend upon

(a) the stage of their condition

(b) how well they will understand, and

(c) how well they might cope with the news.

I think that on the whole *early* diagnosis is the key here, for that allows much more frank and collaborative discussions with the individual concerned.

The situation was summarised by one person in this way:

> This is a thorny issue. Whilst I agree in principle that everyone has the right to know their diagnosis, the proviso has to be 'if they want to'. Telling someone who does not want to know may be as harmful as lying to someone who does.
>
> One of the reasons that the diagnosis is not told in our workplace is that our consultant is afraid that the patient will attempt self-harm. In addition, it may be because we want to avoid the potential painful process of disclosure. I would like to see this changed, but not to a *carte blanche* disclosure to every patient irrespective of their wishes. Establishing how much they want to know is difficult and will have to take into account the wishes of the family. We must encourage disclosure rather than discourage it. But, if the family or patient are adamant about not knowing, then we must keep quiet.
>
> As our ability to diagnose earlier increases, so denying patients their diagnosis gets harder, because they are more able to challenge us. I regard this as a positive process. If we could offer better hope of treatment, perhaps we would be happier about revealing diagnosis. Encouraging the development of social and psychological services may go some way to challenging 'therapeutic nihilism' to positive thinking and a greater willingness to discuss diagnosis. We must encourage and become more responsive to the demands of our clients.

The demands of the clients would seem to be moving in the direction of wanting the diagnosis to be shared with them, at the earliest possible opportunity; this was certainly the view expressed by Kennedy and Rossor (1993) who wrote that

> most carers wish retrospectively that the likely diagnosis had been discussed at an earlier stage and some of the likely problems highlighted…a recent meeting for younger onset patients attended by carers and their professional counterparts asked for a better service from both GPs and hospital practitioners – specifically they wanted the diagnosis to be established earlier and the illness discussed in a realistic and understanding fashion. Education about dementia, its causes and prognosis was felt to be a necessary prerequisite, but sadly lacking.

The doctors' dilemma

Alan Jacques (1987), one of the most respected voices in dementia care, wrote that, 'Contact with relatives of dementia sufferers and voluntary groups such as the Alzheimer's Disease Society reveals their deep frustration about the medical profession in general and general practitioners in particular'. Several of the respondents agreed with this view. The secretary of a local Alzheimer's Disease Society virtually echoed Jacques' words:

> I find professionals are very reluctant to be open and honest, and this needs to be addressed very quickly. The type of answer given by a GP, 'Well there is nothing we can do and it's up to you to cope as best you can,' does not prepare people for the traumatic effects of dementia.

Whilst a development officer reflected that, 'response to dementia seems to be changing very slowly but GPs in particular, in my experience, are not adept at handling this sensitively'.

There can be knock-on effects which leave other people feeling unsure of their role, as one social worker explained; 'People are not very honest with people with dementia. It is one of those awful situations where social services do not feel able to tell someone if the doctors haven't...' A speech therapist experienced a similar predicament; 'I feel that it is not my role to inform patients of their diagnosis, and I am guilty of avoiding issues brought up by patients'.

Steve McLean in an 1987 article says that the attitude of general medicine towards people with dementia has been one of neglect, and he tried to tease out why this should be the case. He suggested that the roots of such neglect may well lie in a number of different factors:

- There may be a kind of 'therapeutic nihilism' amongst doctors when they have to deal with chronic and usually progressive illnesses such as those which cause dementia. This phrase owes its origin to work done in 1961, and describes the sense of hopelessness which can confront people who spend their time endeavouring to make people well.

- Work with people with dementia may often be 'unaesthetic, sometimes dirty' and there may be disturbing and intractable behaviour problems. These can combine to make this sort of work appear unattractive to some people.

- Dealing with incurable conditions can be extremely frustrating and 'thwart a doctor's desire to succeed'.

- The work requires that doctors become involved in the emotionally draining distress and pathos that people and their families experience.

- It is more difficult for the doctor to remain 'outside' and professionally distant. McLean describes it as 'the threat to the clinician's sense of invulnerability that comes from dealing with ageing, dying and mentally deteriorating people'.

- Added to all this, the work takes place in a social context which rates work with the elderly low down in terms of status and resource allocation. He says that we live in a society with inherent prejudices against the elderly, which places great stress on youth, fitness and beauty and which devalues the 'no longer productive' elderly – 'discarding them as if they are worn-out consumer disposable products'.

There is evidence to suggest that the climate is gradually changing, and this can be seen from the increased number of books and journal articles related to dementia and the growing number of specialist centres and pieces of research concerned with dementia. However, change comes slowly and its consequences take time to trickle down.

Later in his article McLean turns his attention to the difficulties of diagnosis and he points out that the very nature of dementia makes its clinical features diverse and non-specific. This is a point which several people raised in their comments to me. Making a diagnosis is extremely difficult. Because the illnesses develop gradually, it is very easy to overlook the early symptoms, and it is difficult to assess with much degree of accuracy the date of onset. People are often reluctant to go to a doctor in the early stages, as many people suffering from dementia are reasonably fit in their body in the early stages of the illness and so it is often impossible to get them to attend a surgery. This means that the chances of making an early diagnosis are considerably reduced. It is also true that the boundaries between a normal ageing process and dementia are often quite blurred. Dementia is not part of the normal ageing process, it is related to a quite specific illness or illnesses, but the early manifestations of that illness may be remarkably similar to normal ageing. Thus the particular illness may be quite advanced before it is clear that this is not normal ageing but a form of dementia. There is considerable reluctance on the part of many GPs, if not most, to test for dementia (O'Connor et al. 1993), and so it would appear that a great many people fail to have an accurate diagnosis and are left to think that 'problems with their memory' are a consequence of their advancing years. Dementia is also difficult to diagnose because there are several other medical conditions which can present identical or similar symptoms, 'thus masquerading as dementia'.

McLean (1987) states that mistakes of three kinds can often be seen in clinical practice, and these have been identified and verified in a number of studies. He groups the mistakes as overdiagnosis, missed diagnosis and misdiagnosis.

Overdiagnosis is what happens when people with a non-dementing illness are diagnosed as having dementia. Many studies have been made in this area, and McLean concluded that in the fourteen different studies that he looked at it appeared that there was an overall misdiagnosis in 15 per cent of the patients diagnosed as having dementia, and whilst he could raise certain methodological questions about some of the studies, nevertheless 'a relatively high rate of overdiagnosis has been consistently demonstrated...and it highlights the need for careful and comprehensive assessment before labelling any person as "demented"' (p.146).

Missed diagnosis also seems to be a common occurrence and McLean says that

> families often find a lack of interest when doctors are consulted about memory loss and other manifestations of dementia. They complain that getting any diagnosis made is more often a problem than misdiagnosis or overdiagnosis. (p.146)

He goes on to quote Berkowitz (1981) who claimed that most doctors are unaware of dementing syndromes and the importance of recognising cognitive impairment in elderly people. Studies provide 'firm evidence' to suggest that doctors in everyday practice often fail to recognise dementia and there is a great need for them to assess the mental state of all elderly patients. An article in the BMJ in 1988 (O'Connor *et al.* 1988) suggested that GPs were more likely to detect dementia in patients that they saw regularly than in those whom they saw infrequently. If this is the case, then it is all the more important that use is made of standard testing procedures, as the opportunities for missing a diagnosis obviously multiply the less well-known a patient is.

Misdiagnosis is when people who have dementia are initially diagnosed as suffering from something else. Confusion is often caused by the manner in which patients present themselves. Depression, anxiety or delirium are often discussed in these early consultations, and studies show that many people are treated for something other than dementia because their symptoms are difficult to isolate and understand. It is important to remember that dementia itself is not an illness but a syndrome – a name given to a cluster of different illnesses which produce certain distinguishing symptoms. The general practitioner is not therefore looking for one particular illness called dementia, but for one of a variety of illnesses most of which are extremely difficult to diagnose.

All this helps us to understand just what a difficult job the general practitioner has when trying to make a diagnosis. If we also realise that the average consultation time is about five minutes (Sutcliffe 1990), and that before the 1980s the topic of dementia was virtually ignored in standard medical texts so that many GPs did not even study it during their training, then we can see that there really is something of a dilemma for many of them. This was a theme that received a wide coverage in the responses that I received. One person summed up the situation in this way:

> I have found that a high proportion of informal carers have not been given a diagnostic label for the condition afflicting their relative. I would enter a caveat however, from a research perspective but one which also applies to care services. I think a description of the symptoms such as 'problems with your memory' is appropriate when it is not known to the worker (or researcher) (a) if a diagnosis has been made or (b) if that diagnosis has been communicated to the person in question.

> A diagnosis of dementia is not something to be made lightly and it must be made by referral to an appropriate specialist. I am as concerned that some people may be wrongly labelled as having dementia (and possibly 'written off' as a result) as I am that many people are not given a label for their problem.

> Withholding information (e.g. a diagnosis) is generally unacceptable (though there can be times when it is the least harmful course of action), but so too is filling an information 'gap' when one is not the appropriate person to do so. The buck lies with the medical profession, and specifically with psychogeriatricians and general practitioners.

One interesting development in recent years has been the setting up of Memory Clinics which can help in diagnosing and providing support for the management of dementia. Marion McMurdo (1993) writes of the Dundee clinic:

> It is a regrettably common experience that patients with dementing illnesses present to the hospital services at an advanced stage of their illness. This often coincides with a domestic crisis, when the patience of unsupported carers and neighbours is at an end. In recognition of this unsatisfactory state of affairs, Memory Clinics were set up in the USA and later in the UK...the aim of a Memory Clinic is to offer an

accessible and acceptable service to those for whom forgetfulness is a problem.

Our experience confirms that of others, that a Memory Clinic is an effective way of finding patients in the early stages of a dementing illness… Another useful function of the clinic is to detect potentially remediable causes of forgetfulness. Of our first fifty patients, eight were suffering from a treatable psychiatric disorder (anxiety or depression). Perhaps disappointingly, only three patients were considered to have a reversible organic disorder…these patients have been reassured and the clinic has hopefully removed the spectre of dementia from them…one aspect of the clinic which is particularly appreciated by the GP colleagues is the multidisciplinary nature of the assessment. (pp.203, 205)

The issue of communication

Given all these difficulties, just how are people diagnosed and how is the news given to them? There seems to be extraordinary diverse practice here. But for those of us who are involved in the ongoing care of people with dementia it is important that we know what the person has been told, the extent to which they have understood (or still do understand) what they were told, and the extent to which their principal informal carers and family know and understand what is happening.

A lady I was speaking to recently was most distressed as her husband had been ill for over six years and she had never been given a diagnosis. There was a mixture of anger and guilt as she battled on, wondering why no diagnosis was given and unsure of the steps that she should be taking. 'If only I knew,' was a constant refrain. Her response to her husband's condition was one of caring for a person with dementia, and she was plugged into various forms of social support, but she desperately wanted some form of confirmation from her GP and this was not forthcoming.

It would be helpful if we were more aware of how diagnoses are shared. Is it with the person himself or herself alone, or together with their family? Some people seem to share the diagnosis with the family but not with the person. Sometimes it is given at one session and sometimes it is spread over several meetings. Sometimes (usually?) it is verbal, but sometimes it is accompanied with written notes and with helpful supplementary booklets and information sheets. Sometimes the diagnosis is not given until there is evidence of social and psychological support structures, and sometimes it is given without them and seemingly with little commitment to provide them.

It would also be helpful if we had more knowledge about how the information is received by people, the extent of their understanding, and their methods of understanding it and coming to terms with it. Some of the interviews I conducted with over 70 carers whilst working on another project showed that most people did not receive information about dementia (at least in terms of understanding it) from their GP, but from television programmes, magazine and newspaper articles and from conversations with friends. More detailed understanding came from subsequently attending support group meetings for carers.

Perhaps it is fitting that a final comment should come from two people who have the responsibility for talking to people about their diagnosis. A consultant in the psychiatry of old age wrote:

> I agree in principle with all your key statements except for number ten, where I feel that there remains sufficient uncertainty about prognosis and reliability of the diagnosis in very early dementia to make it a very different condition from cancer. Honesty is all very well but at times the uncertainties we face are very difficult to adequately convey. However much I might try to convey this I cannot escape the fact that patients consulting me expect me to be authoritative when the reality is often that I don't know... I have numerous examples from clinical practice usually where I am stumped for a solution to the patient until I sit down and communicate properly with them – at which point they may suggest the solution themselves.

And from the Internet, where there was quite a discussion taking place about the problems of diagnosing Alzheimer's disease, an American contributor offered this:

> I'll try to summarize my own approach as a physician.
>
> (a) The patient with a diagnosis of probable Alzheimer's disease (or any other dementia, for that matter) should be told the diagnosis by their physician – even though the AD sufferer may forget. This is *not* a job that should be dumped on the family. (I do not think it is fair to put family members in the position of 'delivering' the news – doing so tends to direct hostility and frustration towards family members, undermining their closeness to the patient and increasing suffering to all).
>
> (b) Unless so demented that the patient cannot really make his/her views known about treatments, research studies, resuscitation status, terminal care etc. I think every AD victim has a right to

know the diagnosis. Otherwise, that individual is robbed of the chance to determine or help determine their own future.

(c) The diagnosis is best approached gradually, with repetition – starting with the information that AD is a consideration in evaluating memory problems in the elderly (most patients already know this), to an eventual discussion of the clinical diagnosis of probable AD and its therapeutic and prognostic implications. That is, one does not see a patient, say 'you have probable Alzheimer's' and goodbye.

(d) When the diagnosis is presented, a therapeutic and management plan should be explained, and alternatives presented.

(e) We provide written notes at the time the diagnosis is formalised, so that the patient and their family members (assuming any are involved, which is not always the case) can refer back to this when something is forgotten or an argument arises ('I just have a little memory problem, nothing that should keep me from driving...').

(f) Follow-up availability of health professionals to answer questions, treat reactive depression etc. is also important...the public perception of AD as being only end-stage dementia is hard to overcome (as old memories are better preserved) – but there clearly is quite a spread. The diagnosis can be made reasonably accurately in patients who are quite capable of understanding the diagnosis.

Enough logorrhea for now – I hope this is of some help.

CHAPTER 14

A Reflective Conclusion[1]

To what extent is it possible to hear the voice of people with dementia? To what extent are they able to reflect upon what is happening to them? How much do we know about what is going on inside a person's brain and personality, and how their illness is affecting their perceptions and their evaluating processes?

The following was found in a gentleman's possessions when his home was being cleared out after his admission into residential care. It is reproduced just as he wrote it. It is obvious that he had been reflecting and writing, trying to make sense of his condition, but increasingly finding that his world was narrowing and his options becoming more limited. But he was aware, and he was concerned, and he was endeavouring to communicate that concern.

> I feel that I am slowly becoming
> 'uncertain', I forget things, times, people
> I am not sure what I should do.
> I discovered a place where I could buy
> things…but have forgotten where it is.
> I am afraid to go ahead and do things.
> As I write at the window I am not sure
> where the road, left or write, goes. Opposite
> to me is a man who has sat opposite me
> for many, many times…but I don't know
> his name, I think it is Sunday, I am
> not sure if I should go to church.
> I *think* Alison is coming after lunch
> to take me to their house – There are

---

1   Much of this chapter has also appeared in an issue of *Findings* published by the Joseph Rowntree Foundation.

children at the house: I know them
but I am not sure what they will be
doing.
'Uncertainty' is not the same as 'madness'
but it is groying that way. I can talk
about things & people but it is very
much a cover-up, and I don't follow
it up

An interesting correspondence, or perhaps conversation would be a better word, was conducted on the Internet, the developing art of communicating worldwide by means of computers. A carer in the United States had this to say:

> Over the past weekend, I lost my favourite patient. He was a wonderful 68 year-old man who was in the very last stages of the disease. I was very close to him because many times I was the only one who could calm him down when he was agitated. I took care of him for a year and watched his condition progress rapidly.
>
> Although he was for the most part unable to communicate his thoughts and ideas, I always felt that he was in there somewhere because I could see the gentleness in his eyes and the warmth when I would hold his hand.
>
> There were a few occasions over the year that he was with us when he would have a very clear day and say some amazing things to me. One day he came up to me and told me he didn't know what to do because he was losing his brain. This was the first time I ever heard him say anything to the effect that he knew what was happening to him. I just held his hand and told him that I loved him and that I would help him through. He smiled at me and told me he loved me. Then two minutes later he was off in another world again. ...One thing that is comforting to me is that he was allowed to die with dignity, and this is a big issue with me. He was thrown out of other facilities and nursing homes because they couldn't handle his behaviours. We are trained to deal with these behaviours and we never drug our patients if at all possible. If he had been in another facility he would have most likely have been drugged and restrained. Instead, he was allowed to die naturally, in his sleep. I only wish it could be this way for all Alzheimer's disease patients. They are often misunderstood.

They are often misunderstood – this is at the heart of communication, and this book, the result of my own particular project, has been concerned with facilitating communication, helping to remove misunderstanding, facilitating the voice of the person with dementia to be heard and encouraged those involved in that process.

The 1990 NHS and Community Care Act requires service providers to consult with their consumers about the services they would wish to receive. In the field of dementia care, the carer has been perceived as being the consumer. This view is now being questioned. In order to improve services for people with dementia and to make them more responsive to individual need it is necessary first to accept that they have a voice, second to facilitate the use of that voice, and third to hear it.

It is only relatively recently that informal carers, usually family members, have been recognised by professionals as partners in the process of caring for people with dementia. The next stage in this process is to admit that the person with dementia is also a partner. We need to find ways of communicating with them and discovering their views on the services which are, or should be, provided.

Communication is possible

Communication is possible, although it is often a difficult and complex process. There is often a great deal of metaphor and symbolism used in speech. There are may nonverbal ways in which communication can take place, and these need to be explored and understood, as do the varying techniques of verbal communication.

We have evidence of people in advanced states of dementia being able to express preferences and reflect subjectively. A desire for widespread training in communication approaches and techniques was raised time and again during this project by people involved in providing care.

Community Care is based on the view that people can make informed choices; if people with dementia do not, then it raises questions about the underlying philosophy. Many services though seem to expect people with dementia *not* to have a voice and this reflects on the failure of current practice to reach people with dementia. To think that they *can* have a voice is to suggest that the culture of care is in need of change.

Challenging behaviour

When people are not 'heard' they may become irritable or aggressive and often they pose the greatest difficulties for staff providing services. Three things seem to be needed:

(a) a greater understanding of *why* people behave in the way that they do

(b) a better understanding of our *own* reactions to challenging behaviour, and how we cope with these, and

(c) more information and understanding about possible ways of handling and interpreting such behaviour.

We need to develop a mindset which is always looking for explanations, for there is invariably a reason for any behaviour. Challenging behaviour is likely to be an expression of fear, anger or frustration. It may also be a valid response to the way that the world is perceived by the person with dementia. As yet we know little about the ways in which they interpret their immediate world.

Behaviour is often interpreted as being aggressive (which it may, or may not be) and it can be frightening; but some people become withdrawn or make no demands, and they too need to be understood. There may be a number of reasons for challenging behaviour apart from the specific demanding illness.

Drug treatment should be the last resort when working with people whose behaviours may be difficult or disruptive. People responding to this project often urged that *understanding and interpreting* behaviour was more important than *managing and controlling it.*

People are affected in different ways
Whilst access to most services is dependent upon a diagnosis of 'dementia', that is not always a straightforward process. It is increasingly being argued that we should understand dementia as a complex interaction between personality, age, biography, ethnicity, health, gender, neurological impairment and the social psychology and web of relationships that a person has. This is to move away from an overemphasis upon a biomedical model and to recognise that we need to treat people as unique individuals.

Many services now work towards creating individualised care plans, but there is often a discrepancy between what is the general policy and what actually happens. Also, such care plans are often problem-centred, highlighting what a person *cannot* do rather than what they are still able to achieve. Given that everyone has an individual pathway through the disease, we need to know them really well, and this knowledge should be reflected in their care plan.

The pace and 'world' of the person with dementia

There is a real danger that people with dementia will lose out in the present system of health care and social provision because communicating with them invariably takes time. It is a process which cannot be rushed, and to try to 'quicken things along' is invariably counter-productive. If we are serious about hearing their voice and seeking their views then we must be prepared to work at their pace and enter into their 'world'. This is extremely difficult when the pressures that drive our current services are those which tend to negate the time and pace which people recognise as being essential.

Pleas for more time to listen and to respond appropriately came from all the sectors involved in this project. Perhaps there is a place here for appropriately trained volunteers. What is quite clear is that *busy professionals with targets to meet and diaries to keep are less likely to be able to hear the voice of people with dementia than those who have the time and skill to adjust their pace and mindset.*

Service planners, managers, purchasers and providers have a responsibility to ensure that every effort has been made to ease the process of communication. So often this is not the case, and the onus is placed on the person with dementia who is then deemed to be 'unable to communicate'.

The impact of the environment

People's ability to communicate, whether at home or in residential care, may be affected by the time of day, the location, background noises, the colour of the flooring or walls, the intensity of lighting or by their general fatigue. Failure to communicate at one particular time and place may not mean that a person is unable to communicate.

Design is very influential and should help to enable rather than disempower people even further. Attention needs to be given, for instance, to the number of 'decision points' a person has to pass and the ways in which signs and labels are devised and placed.

One manger of service commented:

> this might seem a daft thing to say but is it not common sense to assume that by removing someone from their home and placing them in a strange ward, full of strange people and routines, to assess their level of confusion, you will discover a very very confused person.

Many respondents in the project wrote of their near desperation at not being able to provide the sort of service they wanted to. Some of the frustrations were complex and costly, but far too many were straightforward – such as problems inadequate hearing aids, spectacles, painful feet or ill-fitting dentures attended to. The comment was made that is appears to be much easier for a person with dementia to be provided with a nice deep armchair (difficult to get out of!) than for these other factors to be dealt with.

The need for early diagnosis

If people do not know what they are suffering from and what the possible development of their illness might be, then how realistic is it to ask if they are satisfied with the services they are receiving? Far too many people are not diagnosed until a relatively late stage in their illness by which time, for many of them, it is too late to make appropriate plans or to let their wishes be known. It then becomes a difficult and complex task to elicit information; given an earlier diagnosis it would almost certainly have been simpler.

There is a deep frustration amongst carers and service providers about the lateness of most diagnoses. GPs point to the difficulties inherent in making a definite diagnosis, the differing abilities of people to accept what must, inevitably, be bad news, and the lack of information about and availability of appropriate back-up services.

Many people with dementia, carers, and service providers feel that they have been undermined and disempowered by professionals not being honest with them. *Providing an accurate diagnosis, which people are able to understand, and providing supportive structures which enable people to talk with each other and with those who are responsible for service provision, might be the single most important improvement that can be made in the short-term for people with dementia.*

A skilful task

There are two common misapprehensions when discussing the voice of the people with dementia. One is that you cannot communicate with them because the nature of their illness means that they are unable to reflect or communicate. The second is that we know what they want to communicate, and without realising it, slant or coax or ask leading questions so that people with dementia who are more influenced by feelings than by facts will give the answers which they perceive we want them to give. Ascertaining their views can be a very demanding and skilful job and those who have the responsibility for doing it need a great deal of empathy and training. As things are at the moment, the people with the most time and the greatest opportunities to do this tend to be the least trained and the least influential in making decisions about services.

If we are to discover and hear the voice of people with dementia, then whatever our professional basis, we are confronted by a very difficult and complex tasks. Our failure to master that task can easily give rise to the simple assertion that people with dementia are not able to express a preference or a view.

It is possible to be involved in meaningful communication with the vast majority of people with dementia *but* we must be able to enter into their world, understand their sense of pace and time, recognise the problems of distraction and realise that there are many ways in which people express themselves, and *it is our responsibility* to learn how to recognise these. Our normal professional qualifications and our usual work practices seldom equip us for this task, but it is a voice that is quite literally crying out to be heard.

Hearing the Views
of People with Dementia
A Consultative Discussion Paper

In an attempt to improve services for people with dementia and to make services more flexible and responsive to individual need, we must first accept the premise that people with dementia have a voice that can be heard. This voice may be exhibited in a variety of ways and it is a challenge for all service providers to interpret and facilitate this voice, to hear it, to understand it and to act upon it.

For the past nine months I have been actively involved, within the Dementia Services Development Centre, in exploring potential responses to this challenge and discovering positive ways in which service providers may best hear this voice. Funded by the Joseph Rowntree Foundation, I have undertaken an extensive literature review on this area, held a number of interviews with people with dementia to explore their service needs and liaised closely with key people in the field.

From this initial consultative foundation I have identified 10 themes or key areas on which I would invite **your comments and responses** in relation to facilitating the views, and the voice of people with dementia. This voice needs to be heard and it is our belief, within the Centre, that the wider the consultation, the more representative will be the findings of this study – hence I also need to hear your voice and learn from your experience.

I would be happy for this document to be photocopied and passed on to other people, and I hope that you will be willing to share in this consultative process.

Malcolm Goldsmith
Research Fellow

How to respond to this document

I have identified 10 key issues and briefly expanded the overall theme. Then, in italics, I have suggested one or two questions which might be raised – these are largely for illustrative purposes. Basically I am asking

- Do you agree with the statement?
- Have you any examples to illustrate them, and
- What implications for service provision do they have?

The 10 Key Areas that we would like your views on

1. Communication with people with dementia is possible

It is possible, but it can be a difficult and slow process, requiring time, patience, skill and commitment. If communication is possible, then it must be possible to communicate about services, and for the majority of people with dementia it must be possible for them to communicate their satisfaction (or dissatisfaction) with the services provided. Not to pursue the task of eliciting such views is tantamount to saying either that they are unable to communicate or that their views are irrelevant to service providers.

- *Do you have any experience, suggestions or advice to offer which might help to emphasise this conviction?*

2. The experience of dementia is extremely disempowering

Not only are people having to cope with a debilitating illness, they are also confronted by a plethora of services and service providers. In this process they are often made 'objects' and their dignity and sense of worth is diminished. There is a process of disempowering and disregarding, within which the failure to hear the voice of the person with dementia is one of the most persistent.

- *Have you any examples of the ways in which people with dementia have been empowered? Are there any ways in which service providers can become more aware of this issue and listen to the voice of the people with dementia? What might be the implications for service provision of empowering people?*

3. Different people are affected in different ways

Because people are different, they need to be understood and approached in different ways. It has been argued that dementia is the result of a complex interaction between personality, biography, physical health, neurological impairment and social psychology. Lumping people together under the label of 'dementia' and approaching them in the same way is likely to increase the problems of communication and make it more difficult for us to hear their voice.

   o   *Do you have any experience of treating people in different ways? Have you any suggestions as to how service provision might be more adaptable to differing types of people and illness?*

4. Communication with people with dementia requires respect for their sense of time and pace

Often, difficulties encountered when communicating can be attributed to the pace of the interaction. Communicating with a person with dementia can be a slow process. We must be prepared to devote an adequate and appropriate amount of time to this task. Very often metaphors may be used, which need to be interpreted. Not having enough time, and therefore making little progress, is not the same as saying that the person is unable to communicate. Communication may be extremely difficult because, for whatever reason, we are not able to devote an adequate amount of time to that specific task.

   o   *In your experience, have pressures of time made it more difficult for you to communicate? Have you any suggestions to make as to how service providers can reach a balance between respecting the time and pace of the person with dementia whilst at the same time providing an economical service?*

5. Knowing a person's 'life story' can be an aid to communication

Communication is often assisted by rooting it within the life-context and history of the person with dementia, and in this way it is often possible to discover their views and preferences. Ability to communicate may be related to their ability to communicate before they had dementia. We need to know about their earlier personality and approach to life. Good dementia care is related to the whole person and not just to the 'area of need'.

   o   *Have you any insights to share as to how service provision might be affected if we could set our communication within the life-context of the person with dementia?*

6. Environmental and other factors have an affect upon the process of communicating with people with dementia

The ability of a person with dementia is considerably influenced by a number of environmental factors such as

> location
> the time of day
> background noises
> colour
> the intensity of lighting, and
> general fatigue.

It also seems to be related to the nature of the relationship that the person has with whoever is providing the service or is talking with them.

> ○ *Have you any experience of changes taking place when any of these variables have changed? In what ways do you think we could take these factors more seriously in our work?*

7. There are nonverbal ways in which people with dementia communicate

Many people now find that it is possible to gain an insight into the views and preferences, the mood and sense of well-being of people with dementia through art, music, and different forms of touch. People who find verbal expression difficult invariably find other ways in which to communicate.

> ○ *What has been your experience of nonverbal communication with people with dementia? Do you think that such an approach might be able to improve or enrich your own work? What might be required of your service if it were to concentrate more on nonverbal forms of communication.*

8. 'Challenging behaviour' is a form of communication

We know that people's behaviour, whatever form it takes, is very often an attempt to express something which they are unable to articulate verbally. For instance, wandering or shouting may not simply be a function of the illness. People with dementia may be trying to express their feelings by behaviour patterns which we find difficult to understand or cope with.

> ○ *Can you share how you might have learned to accept such behaviour and tried to interpret it? In what ways might we understand behaviour which we find difficult so as to be able to respond creatively to it?*

9. Group work may help people with poor communication abilities

Even when communication seems very difficult, it is sometimes possible to encourage and stimulate people with dementia in such a way as to facilitate conversation and to discover views and preferences. Sometimes in such a process restless behaviour is reduced and a sense of well-being seems to increase. Some imaginative work has been done with people in small groups, and some people have found ways of encouraging people to set their own agendas in such groups.

> ○ *Do you have any experience of working with people in small groups in ways which enable them to develop their own themes and express their feelings? Have you found ways of helping people with dementia to talk to each other? Do you have experience of working with people in later stages of the illness in this way? In your situation might there be times when a new approach to group work might need to be tried?*

10. People with dementia should be given an open, honest and understandable diagnosis as soon as possible

If people do not know what is wrong with them, and what the development of their illness is likely to be, how realistic is it to ask if they are satisfied with the services being provided? Might they want different services if they knew more about their condition? In my experience very few people seem to have been told or understood their diagnosis or condition and great collusion takes place to ensure that the word 'dementia' is not mentioned. The phrase 'problems with your memory' euphemistically covers known diagnoses. The situation with dementia seems to be where the situation with cancer was twenty years ago.

> ○ *How honest are we in our dealings with people? How do we handle the thorny questions relating to colluding with the avoidance of truth? How are we able to explore the reality of dementia with people and integrity if we are not allowed to discuss the illness? How are people to express their views if they do not know what is wrong with them?*

I hope that you will feel able to respond to this document and thus share in this project – the aim of which is to improve services for people with dementia by finding ways in which we are better able to hear what they have to say, and incorporate their preferences and wishes into the services which they receive. Thank you.

References

Akerlund, B.M. and Norberg, A. (1986) 'Group psychotherapy with demented patients.' *Geriatric Nursing*, March/April.

Allan, K. (1994) 'Dementia in acute units: wandering.' *Nursing Standard 9*, 8.

Allison, A. (1994) 'Dementia in acute units: the issues.' *Nursing Standard 8*, 52.

Archibald, C. (1994) *Sexuality and Dementia*. University of Stirling: Dementia Services Development Centre.

BBC radio discussion (1994) *All in the mind*.

Beattie, A. (1974) 'Errand into the maze: the experience of corridors in hospitals.' *Journal of Architectural Research 3* (2), 44–48.

Beck, Modlin, Heithoff and Shue (1992) 'Exercise as an intervention for behaviour problems.' *Geriatric Nursing*, Sept/Oct.

Bell, N. (1992) *Pink Doors and Door Knockers*. University of Stirling: Dementia Services Development Centre.

Berkowitz, H. (1981) 'House officers' knowledgeability of organic brain syndromes.' *General Hospital Psychiatry 3*.

Booth, T. quoted by A. Butler (1990) 'Research Ethics and Older People in Researching Social Gerontology.' In S. Pearce *Researching Social Gerontology*. London: Sage.

Bowlby, J. (1988) *A Secure Base; Clinical Applications of Attachment Theory*. London: Tavistock/Routledge.

Burley, R. and Pollock, R. (1992) *Every House you'll Ever Need: Designing out Disorientation in the Home*. University of Stirling: Dementia Services Development Centre.

Carr, J. (1995) *Evening Care Project: Valley House, Cowdenbeath*. University of Stirling: Dementia Services Development Centre.

Cobban, N. (1994) *Carpets: A Matter of Opinion*. University of Stirling: Dementia Services Development Centre.

Cohen, D. (1991) 'The subjective experience of Alzheimer's Disease: the anatomy of an illness as perceived by patients and families.' *American Journal of Alzheimer's Care and Related Disorders and Research*, May/June.

Cohen, D. and Eisdorfer (1986) *The Loss of Self: A Family Resource for the Care of Alzheimer's Disease and Related Disorders*. New York: Norton.

Cotrell and Lein (1993) 'Awareness and denial in the Alzheimer's disease victim.'
    Journal of Gerontological Social Work 19, 3/4.

Cotrell, V. and Schulz, R. (1993) 'The perspective of the patient with Alzheimer's
    disease; a neglected dimension of dementia research.' *The Gerontologist 33*, 2.

Crimmens, P. (1994) 'Drama therapy in the care of people with dementia.' Paper
    given at the 1994 Alzheimer's Disease International Conference in Edinburgh.

Crisp, J. (1993) 'Making Sense of what People with Alzheimer's say.' Paper presented
    to Alzheimer's Association of Australia conference on 'Quality of Life', May.

Davis, R. (1989) *My Journey into Alzheimer's Disease.* Amersham: Scripture Press.

De Luca, C. (1995) unpublished.

Department of Health (1992) *The Health of the Nation.* London: HMSO.

Downs, M., Carr, J., Chapman, A., Dunlop, A., Goldsmith, M., McLennan, J. and
    Murphy, C. (1994) *Dementia: A Literature Review for the Northern Ireland Dementia
    Policy Scrutiny.* University of Stirling: Dementia Services Development Centre.

Dunlop, A. (1994) *Hard Architecture and Human Scale Designing for Disorientation.*
    University of Stirling: Dementia Services Development Centre.

Foley, J.M. (1992) 'The experience of being demented.' Binstock, Post and
    Whitehead (eds) *Dementing and Aging: Ethics, Values and Policy Choices.* Baltimore,
    MD: John Hopkins University Press.

Fontana and Smith (1989) 'Alzheimer's disease victims; the "unbecoming" of self and
    the normalization of competence.' *Sociological Perspectives 32*, 1.

Ford, Fox, Fitch and Donovan (1986) 'Light in the darkness.' *Nursing Times*, January 7.

Froggatt, A. (1988) *Self-awareness in Early Dementia. Mental Health Problems in Old Age: A
    Reader.* Milton Keynes: The Open University.

Gibson, F. (1991) 'The Lost Ones: Recovering the past to help their present.' A paper
    given at a BASW study day in Belfast and subsequently published by University of
    Stirling: Dementia Services Development Centre.

Gibson, F. (1994) 'Reading around...reminiscence.' *Journal of Dementia Care*,
    May/June.

Gillies, B. (1995) *The Subjective Experience of Dementia: A Qualitative Analysis of Interviews
    with Dementia Sufferers and Their Carers and the implications for service provision.*
    University of Dundee: Department of Medicine.

Goldsmith, M. and Wharton, M. (1993) *Knowing Me Knowing You.* London: SPCK.

Griffiths, H. (1991) 'The psychiatry of old age: the effects of dementia on
    communication.' In R. Gravell and J. France (eds) *Speech and Communication Problems
    in Psychiatry.* London: Chapman and Hall.

Hamilton, H.E. (1994) *Conversations with an Alzheimer's Patient.* Cambridge: Cambridge
    University Press.

Helen (1994) Printed in the July magazine of the Alzheimer's Association (USA), the
    Cleveland Area Chapter.

Heywood, B. (1994) *Caring for Maria.* Shaftesbury: Element.

Hillan, E. (1993) 'Nursing dementing elderly people: ethical issues.' *Journal of Advanced Nursing 18.*

Holden, U. (1994) 'Dementia in acute wards: aggression.' *Nursing Standard 37,* Dec 7, 9, 11.

Holden, U.P. and Woods, R.T. (1988) *Reality Orientation: Psychological Approaches to the 'Confused' Elderly.* Edinburgh: Churchill Livingstone.

Hussian, R. (1982) 'Stimulus control in the modification of problematic behaviour in elderly institutionalized patients.' *International Journal of Behavioral Geriatrics I,* 33–42.

Jacques, A. (1987) 'Strengthening the primary team in support of dementia sufferers.' *Geriatric Medicine,* November.

Jacques, A. (1992) *Understanding Dementia.* Edinburgh: Churchill Livingstone (Adapted from Jorm (1990)).

Jenny, S. (1994) *Memories in the Making; a Program of Creative Art Expression for Alzheimer's Patients.* California: Alzheimer's Association of Orange County.

Jones, G. (1992) 'A communication model for dementia.' In *Care Giving in Dementia, Research and Application.* London: Tavistock/Routledge.

Kantrowitz, B. (1989) 'Trapped inside her own world.' *Newsweek* Dec 18.

Keady, J., Nolan, M. and Gilliard, J. (1995) 'Listen to the voices of experience.' *Journal of Dementia Care,* May/June.

Kelly, M. (1993) *Designing for People with Dementia in the Context of the Building Standards.* University of Stirling: Dementia Services Development Centre.

Kennedy, A. and Rossor, M. (1993) 'Management of dementia.' *The Practitioner,* February, 237.

Killick, J. (1994) 'Giving shape to shadows.' *Elderly Care 6,* 3, May/June. (See also his *The Times of our Lives* (1994) published by Westminster Health Care, and *Please Give me Back my Personality* (1994) published by University of Stirling: Dementia Services Development Centre.)

Kitwood, T. (1990) 'Psychotherapy and Dementia'. BPS Psychotherapy section newsletter 8.

Kitwood, T. (1990a) 'The dialectics of dementia: with particular reference to Alzheimer's disease.' *Ageing and Society 10.*

Kitwood T. (1993) *Frames of reference for an understanding of dementia.* University of Bradford: Bradford Dementia Research Group.

Kitwood, T. (1993a) 'Discover the person, not the disease.' *Journal of Dementia Care 1,* 1, Nov/Dec.

Kitwood, T. (1993b) 'Towards a theory of dementia care: the interpersonal process.' *Ageing and Society 13.*

Kitwood, T. and Benson, S. (1995) *The New Culture of Dementia Care.* London: Hawker Publications.

Kitwood, T. and Bredin, K. (1992) 'Towards a theory of dementia care: personhood and well-being.' *Journal of the Centre for Policy on Aging and the British Society of Gerontology.*

Lam and Beech (1994) 'I'm Sorry to go Home: The Weekend Break Project: Consultation with Users and Their Carers.' Monograph from Department of Psychology, St Helier NHS Trust, Sutton Hospital, Cotswold Road, Sutton, Surrey SM2 5NF.

Lee, V. (1991) 'Language changes in Alzheimer's disease: A literature review.' *Journal of Gerontological Nursing 17*, 1.

Li, C.K. (1993) 'On listening to the patient.' *Clinical Psychology Forum 62.*

Lubinski, R. (1991) *Dementia and Communication.* London: Decker.

Lyman, K. (1989) 'Bringing the social back in: A critique of the biomedicalization of dementia.' *The Gerontologist 29*, 5.

McGahan, A. (1994) 'The difficulties of diagnosis in the early stages.' *Issues in Focus.* Alzheimer's Association, Cleveland Area Chapter (USA) July.

McGowin, D. (1993) *Living in the Labyrinth: a Personal Journey Through the Maze of Alzheimer's.* San Fransisco: Elder Books.

McGregor, I. and Bell, J. (1993) 'Voyage of discovery.' *Nursing Times 89*, 36.

McGregor, I. and Bell, J. (1994) 'Buzzing with life, energy and drive.' *Journal of Dementia Care 2*, 6.

McLean, S. (1987) 'Assessing dementia part 1: difficulties, definitions and differential diagnosis.' *The Australian and New Zealand Journal of Psychology 21*, 142–174.

McMurdo, M., Grant, D., Gilchrist, J., Findlay, D., McLennan, J. and Lawrence, B. (1993) 'The Dundee Memory Clinic: the first 50 patients.' *Health Bulletin 51*, 4, July.

Marshall, M. (1993) in the Introduction to *Dementia: New Skills for Social Workers.* London: Jessica Kingsley Publishers.

Milke (1992) 'Wandering tracks; environmental strategies that may work too well.' In G. Gutman (ed) *Shelter and Care of Persons with Dementia.* Vancouver: Simon Fraser University.

Mills, M. (1992) 'Dementia, reminiscence, and counselling skills: a new approach?' *Journal of the British Society of Gerontology 2*, 1.

Mills and Chapman (1992) 'Understanding the story.' *Nursing the Elderly 4*, 5.

Mills and Coleman (1994) 'Nostalgic memories in dementia – a case study.' *International Journal of Ageing and Human Development 38*, 3.

Morris, J. (1993) 'Including Older People in Community Care Planning.' In J. Morris and V. Lindlow (1993) *User Participation in Community Care Services.* London: Department of Health.

Murphy, C. (1994) *It Started with a Sea-shell: Life Story Work and People with Dementia.* University of Stirling: Dementia Services Development Centre.

National Consumer Council (1990) *Consulting Consumers in the National Health Service: Services for Elderly People with Dementia Living at Home.* London: National Consumer Council.

Naughtin, G. and Laidler, T. (1991) *When I Grow too Old to Dream.* Victoria: Collins Dove.

O'Connor, Pollitt, P., Hyde, J., Brook, C., Reiss, B. and Roth, M. (1988) 'Do general practitioners miss dementia in elderly patients?' *British Medical Journal 297,* 29 October.

O'Connor, Fertig, A., Grande, M., Hyde, J., Perry, J., Boland, M., Silverman, J. and Wraight, S. (1993) 'Dementia in general practice: the practical consequences of a more positive approach to diagnosis.' *British Medical Journal 302.*

Peloquin, S. (1993a) 'The depersonalization of patients: a profile gleaned from narratives.' *American Journal of Occupational Therapy 47.*

Peloquin, S. (1993b) 'The patient–therapist relationship: beliefs that shape care.' *The American Journal of Occupational Therapy 47.*

Phair, L. (1990) *What the People Think: Homefield Place from the Clients Point of View.* Monograph from Eastbourne and County Healthcare, Seaford Day Hospital, Sutton Road, Seaford, East Sussex.

Pietrukowicz, M. and Johnson, M. (1991) 'Using life histories to individualise Nursing Home staff attitudes towards residents.' *The Gerontologist 31,* 1.

Rau, M.T. (1991) 'Impact on families.' A chapter in Lubinski (1991).

Rau, M.T. (1993) 'Coping With Communication Challenges in Alzheimer's Disease.' *Coping with Aging Series.* San Diego, CA: Singular Publishing Group.

Robinson A., Spencer B. and White L. (1989) *Understanding Difficult Behaviors – some practical suggestions for coping with Alzheimer disease and related illnesses.* Geriatric Education Centre of Michigan, Eastern Michigan University, 416 King Hall, Ypsilanti, Michigan, 48197

Sabat, S. and Harre, R. (1992) 'The construction and deconstruction of self in Alzheimer's disease.' *Ageing and Society 12.*

Sacks, O. (1983) 'Awakenings.' Quoted in Peloquin (1993b).

Sacks, O. (1984) *A Leg to Stand On.* New York: Harper and Row. Quoted in Peloquin (1993a).

Seaman, L. (1982) 'Affective Nursing Touch.' *Geriatric Nursing* May/June.

Senile, Polk, P. (1979–80) In Janeczko *Postcard poems: a collection of poetry for sharing.* New York: Bradbury Press. Quoted in Lee, Virginia (1991); Language changes in Alzheimer's disease: A literature review *Journal of Gerontological Nursing 17,* 1.

Sinason, V. (1992) *Mental Handicap and the Human Condition,* especially the chapter 'The Man Who was Losing His Brain.' London: Free Association Books.

Singer, P. (1994) *Rethinking Life and Death: The Collapse of our Traditional Ethics.* Singapore: Oxford Paperbacks.

Smithers, J. (1977) 'Dimensions of senility.' In *Urban Life 6,* and quoted in Hamilton.

Social Services Inspectorate (1993) *Inspecting for Quality; Standards for the Residential Care of Elderly People with Dementia.* London: HMSO/Department of Health.

Sperlinger and McAuslane (1994) *I Don't Want you to Think I'm Ungrateful...but it Doesn't Satisfy What I Want.* Monograph available from the Department of Psychology, St Helier NHS Trust, Sutton Hospital, Cotswold Road, Sutton, Surrey SM2 5NF.

Spivack, M. (1967) 'Sensory distortions in tunnels and corridors.' *Hospital and Community Psychiatry 18*, 24–30.

Stevens, S., Pitt, B., Nicholl, C., Fletcher, A., and Palmer, A. (1992) 'Language assessment in a memory clinic.' *International Journal of Geriatric Psychiatry 7.*

Sutcliffe, D. (1990) 'Alzheimer's Disease; why the GP may not seem to care.' *Horizons,* May.

Sutton and Fincham (1994) 'Clients' perspectives: experiences of respite care.' *PSIGE Newsletter 49*, March.

Takahiro, S. (1991) *Coping with senile dementia: 12 rules for better nursing care.*

Teri, L., Rabins, P., Whitehouse, P., Berg, L., Reisberg, B., Sunderland, T., Eichelman, B. and Phelps, C. (1992) 'Management of behaviour disturbance in Alzheimer's disease: current knowledge and future direction.' *Alzheimer Disease and Associate Disorders 6*, 2.

Thomas, R.S. (1988) *The Echoes Return Slow.* Chippendale, NSW: Papermac.

Thomas, R.S. (1990) *Counterpoint.* Newcastle Upon Tyne: Bloodaxe Books.

Walker, S. (1988) 'The challenge of dementia – first we need information.' *Speech Therapy in Practice*, March.

Winner, M. (1993) 'User Choice, Care Management and People with Dementia.' A paper given at the British Society of Gerontology Conference.

Wishart, R. (1990) 'When all is lost in the recesses of the mind.' *The Scotsman,* November 6th.

Yale, R. (1993) *Research Summary: Support Groups for Newly Diagnosed, Early Stage Alzheimer's Patients. How patients manage their concerns.*

Yale, R. (1993a) *A Guide to Facilitating Support Groups for Newly Diagnosed Alzheimer's Patients.*

Yale, R. (1993b) 'Contents of patients' concerns in groups.' These are some of a number of papers obtainable from LCS 1067 Filbert Street, Suite 100, San Francisco, California 94133. Other sheets are headed: 'Issues to consider in setting up early stage AD patient support groups'; 'Screening and interviewing patient support group participants'; 'Support groups for early stage Alzheimer's patients – group process issues' and 'Observations of patients' responses to groups.'

Index